THE ROUTLEDGE INTRODUCTION TO CANADIAN LITERATURE AND ILLNESS

The Routledge Introduction to Canadian Literature and Illness considers the key literary and historical frameworks for reading stories about sickness. Transcending disciplinary boundaries, this book analyzes narrative depictions of major epidemics, disastrous injuries, mental and maternal health, medical assistance in dying, and the curative effects of decolonization. This accessible and engaging guide illustrates how illness, encompassing states of physical and mental disorder, injury, and disruption, provides structure and focus to many of the most significant works of English narrative published in Canada. Giving distinct consideration to Indigenous authors who may or may not identify as Canadian and whose representations of illness reflect centuries of colonial violence, this volume offers timely resources to think critically and originally about the Canadian canon for fruitful classroom discussion. Students of both literature and health humanities will find that this book deepens their understanding of literary portrayals of illness and the impact of narrative on concepts of affliction and healing.

Jessica Duffin Wolfe is Professor of Media, Creative Arts, and Design at Humber College. She holds a PhD in English, Book History and Print Culture from the University of Toronto.

Routledge Introductions to Canadian Literature

Series Editors
Robert Lecker, *McGill University*
Lorraine York, *McMaster University*

Routledge Introductions to Canadian Literature is a series that provides critical introductions to important trends, issues, authors, historical, cultural and intellectual contexts in Canadian Literature. The series draws on the work of experts in the field to provide a detailed but accessible commentary on those works or conceptual issues which are taught with undergraduate students in mind but also graduate students and instructors.

The Routledge Introduction to the Canadian Short Story
Maria Löschnigg

The Routledge Introduction to Twentieth- and Twenty-First-Century Canadian Poetry
Erin Wunker

The Routledge Introduction to English Canadian Literature and Digital Humanities
Paul Barrett and Sarah Roger

The Routledge Introduction to Canadian Literature and Illness
Jessica Duffin Wolfe

For more information about this series, please visit: https://www.routledge.com/Routledge-Introductions-to-Canadian-Literature/book-series/RICL

THE ROUTLEDGE INTRODUCTION TO CANADIAN LITERATURE AND ILLNESS

Jessica Duffin Wolfe

Routledge
Taylor & Francis Group
NEW YORK AND LONDON

Designed cover image: Getty Images

First published 2025
by Routledge
605 Third Avenue, New York, NY 10158

and by Routledge
4 Park Square, Milton Park, Abingdon, Oxon, OX14 4RN

Routledge is an imprint of the Taylor & Francis Group, an informa business

ISBN: 978-1-032-37402-4 (hbk)
ISBN: 978-1-032-37401-7 (pbk)
ISBN: 978-1-003-34011-9 (ebk)

DOI: 10.4324/9781003340119

Typeset in Sabon
by Apex CoVantage, LLC

For my parents,
Jacalyn Duffin and Robert David Wolfe

CONTENTS

ACKNOWLEDGEMENTS

Thank you to Robert Lecker and Lorraine York for the invitation to write this book and for their feedback, and to three anonymous readers whose reports also improved these chapters. The lessons of many past teachers, especially Allan Hepburn and Audrey Jaffe, echoed as I worked, while two impromptu parkside advice sessions with Thomas Keymer helped bring this book into being. I relied on the holdings of both Humber Polytechnic and the University of Toronto to complete this work, and on the kindness of the summer staff at the Eberhard Zeidler Library. My students at Humber teach me more about storytelling every day I get to work with them.

Family and friends have offered crucial support and diversions, and I am grateful to Shawn Micallef, Massih Moayedi, Elizabeth Bowie, Claire Taylor Hansen, Rebecca Collard, and Nancy Epstein. My father-in-law, the psychiatrist and author David Goldbloom, shared essential thoughts on the manuscript. Thanks to Kyle Wyatt for many glasses of wine over two decades of friendship and for publishing the essay that prompted this volume, and to Juvelyne Julian for making my home a place I could work. I am grateful to my children, Wolf and Kensington Goldbloom, for the delight they bring to my days, and to Daniel Goldbloom for his faith, jokes, music, and love.

My parents offered vital and tireless encouragement, thoughts, and feedback on this book, and it is dedicated to them in thanks for a lifetime of help, inspiration, reading, and affection. My thoughtful and strategic father, the policy scholar and retired diplomat Robert David Wolfe, makes many adventures possible, and his tasty meals, belief in the importance of literary criticism, and preternaturally sage advice are among the key ingredients of this book. Throughout my childhood, from my first outing at ten days old to a seminar at the Sorbonne, my mother, the hematologist and medical historian Jacalyn Duffin, let me learn at her side in archives across Canada, France, and Italy, and brought me along to conferences from Mexico City to Geneva. As she shared and explained the miracles she witnessed along the path of her scholarship, her intellectual journeys became mine. Without the model of her immense curiosity and attention to suffering, and her willingness and work to bring me along for the ride, this book would not exist.

INTRODUCTION

Narrative Uses of Illness in Canada

This is a book about how illness appears in and impacts the literary stories told by Canadians. In her essay on reading while sick, Virginia Woolf argues that the relative absence of illness in literature is because of its horror: "To look these things squarely in the face," she writes, "would need the courage of a lion tamer; a robust philosophy; a reason rooted in the bowels of the earth" (102). This book aims to look directly at how Canadian authors have looked directly at what it means to be ill.

Whereas "disease" implies a specific biological disorder (Kleinman 3), the varied disruptions of body and mind that I discuss here as "illness" oblige characters to attend to their own suffering and seek help from caregivers. Instead of portraying the full scope of Canadian literary artistry, this book focuses rather narrowly on prose narrative in English to accord with the limits of my own expertise, but also because illness itself is often structured as a story that progresses from stasis to trouble, and sometimes back again. Illness opens narrative avenues for authors and meaning for readers, often beyond a correlation to so-called real life. This book attempts to illustrate such narrative uses of illness through Canadian literary history.

As we shall see in the first chapter on epidemics, illness can let authors stretch the limits of realism or they can use it to put a terminal frame around civilization itself to see and speculate about it more clearly. Disastrous injuries and storytelling caregivers let writers present tenderness towards the past and its stories as reverence for ailing bodies, as we will find in the second chapter. The third chapter considers how stories of mental affliction explore the limits of the mind and communication and illuminate the history of assisted death in Canada, while the fourth chapter

DOI: 10.4324/9781003340119-1

examines pregnancy and birth through novels about their trouble, history, and refusal. The fifth and final chapter looks at how stories about sickness by Indigenous authors depict decolonizing cures.

While the chapters proceed through these topics, I have tried to draw out other relevant themes. Many works discussed here consider the meaning of being a patient and what kind of agency sick people have within the health-care system. Likewise, many of these books examine the often-shifting cultural and practical roles of doctors, nurses, and family members struggling to care for sick loved ones. The meaning of the hospital as a symbol and space that impacts characters' lives and communities recurs in many stories, sometimes set alongside the library as a parallel institution that also ministers to the life and health of the collective. Both spaces circulate information and permit infiltrations and liberties, even as they each restrict and release their occupants. Authors often present nurses in particular as spies, state agents, and gossips, revealing a tacit form of usually feminized power in contrast to the greater official and often-masculinized authority of doctors. Such gender-based disparities denote the historic domination of the practice of medicine by white men.

We will see dualities between mind and body both assumed and denied, the medicalization of fertility, and both venal and altruistic caregivers. These narratives question how and whether healers may accept payment, and whether doing so impacts the quality or legitimacy of their care. These stories ask whether science can harm, and what heals in therapeutic relationships, among friends, loved ones, patients, and medical workers, whether it is treatment that can be swallowed, or whether care itself cures. These texts consider whether caregivers can be trusted to respect boundaries, or to save or end a life when asked. Authors repeatedly question the administration of drugs and other psychotropic or possibly sickening or addictive substances such as alcohol, asking what gets given, by whom, and why, and how social status changes as a result of being a purveyor or consumer of forbidden or curing substances. The added weight literary critics perceive in last or final poems (see Vendler) gives context to stories told by the dying and the elixirs that help draw out their tales in these books. Echoes between diagnosis, narration, and knowledge chime in every chapter, intimating their etymological connections. In these works, medicine can fuel storytelling, even as telling and hearing stories can be a kind of medicine. These throughlines, spurs for narrative, appear throughout the book.

Illness opens gaps in stories and in characters' lives, causing missed chances or making room for illicit encounters and new discoveries. Contagion connects people and causes plot, and lets characters and authors weigh the value of one life against many. Malady in these books invites, excuses, and prevents truth telling, and can cause concealment as well as revelation, memorialization, and supernatural insight. Illness can push characters to find meaning in numbers and lets authors build suspense from counting. Fictional stories of illness can mirror the case studies used in medical education and publication, reflecting overlaps as well as disjunctions in how authors, readers, and the medical profession interpret the meaning of stories. Illness sends characters hunting for causes, and sometimes reveals a pathology in the assumption that disease can be explained. Searching for vocabularies with which to describe chronic suffering, authors question whether, to be an illness, pain must be physical or have a cause and a potential resolution. Authors contrast diagnosis and healing when one should but does not bode the other, and they ask whether the idea of a cure offers false or worthwhile hope. In these books as in medical care, finding the right diagnosis, knowing for example whether someone really needs birth control or antidepressants, depends on the story.

Though narrative can illuminate real suffering, the works assembled here do not perfectly mirror the textured misery Canadians have suffered due to illness over the last two hundred years. In reading for this book, it became clear that, as Woolf predicts, the literary treatments of malady in this country do not precisely document the historical causes of the greatest quotient of death and agony in Canada. Cancer, heart disease, stroke, diabetes, accidental injury, and addiction, along with the physical impacts of poverty, isolation, discrimination, and environmental contamination, would all need to feature more prominently for literature to be representative of Canadians' most statistically prevalent forms of mortal suffering (see Statistics Canada). If narrative does not mirror social reality, it is worth trying to observe what kinds of illness stories do get told, published, and celebrated, and why. If illness in narrative does not reflect contemporaneous struggles, it is serving other functions for authors and for the readers engaged by such stories.

Narrative can be interpreted as an effort to identify and dissipate disorder, so the trouble and disruption of illness offers an ideal frame through which to consider the meaning of storytelling. If fiction explains how individuals change, in stories about sickness, the body and its ailments stand as a proxy for disturbances of character. Sick characters have issues worth fixing, whether they prove intractable, or susceptible to cure, and being ill implies a progression that can shape narrative. Focusing on illness rather than health emphasizes how what's at stake for characters in these stories is their own and others' suffering, sometimes led forward by the prospect of a cure—or just a wish for relief. Illness makes narration matter because it highlights the risk that everyone who could tell a story may die first. The experience draws out fundamental questions about what it means to be alive by forcing the sick to test their footing in the world of the living and consider what might be beyond it. Writing about illness lets authors regard the edges of life, what it means for a person to crumble, to fail and be frail, to be attacked by forces beyond their control, to face their own finitude, and what it means for those around them—beloved, and foe alike—to do the same. Illness stories in general could be said to worry at mortality, seeking to better understand life itself by regarding its borderlands and endings. In narratives of illness, the outcome literally matters, raising both the stakes and the question of what problems storytelling can solve—whether narrative itself can heal.

Despite what Woolf diagnoses as its patchy record of detailed depictions, illness does have a long presence in literature, as I discuss in the essay that sparked this volume ("Pandemic"). The experience has had perhaps an even greater hold on the attention of cultural theorists, while narrative itself is of enduring interest to medical workers. In line with the famous examples of Susan Sontag's long essays from the 1970s and 80s on metaphors attached to tuberculosis, cancer, and AIDS, illness has prompted cultural analysis (see Diedrich), theories of writing by the sick (see Frank; Hawkins), and, especially over the last decade, literary studies of its narrative representations (see Hingston; Jurecic; Krienke; Fifield). In the same timeframe the medical interest in storytelling became so widespread as to prompt a 2011 critique (Woods), and comprises accounts of the narrative meaning of illness for patients and caregivers (see Kleinman), medical knowledge and diagnosis as narrative (Hunter; Jutel), the utility of story in medical care (Robertson et al.; Lucius-Hoene et al.), Barrows and Tamblyn's influential "problem-based" approach to medical education published in 1980, and especially Rita Charon's argument for incorporating story in medical care in *Narrative Medicine* (2006).

Embraced as a core branch of the burgeoning field of the health humanities (see Crawford et al.; Bleakly and Nielson), which often concerns the capacity of art and literature to promote wellness, narrative medicine argues for the integration of story in institutional healthcare. As Laura Moss puts it in her lucid 2015 discussion of narrative medicine in relation to fiction, work in the health humanities often seeks to show "how turning to fiction might help point to some of the shortcomings of contemporary medical practice" (6). Yet the corrective benefits of interdisciplinary conversations and exchange go both ways, and literary scholars might likewise aspire to identify points of medical and scientific anachronism and ignorance in the works we study and celebrate.

I have tried to meet this challenge where possible, but my primary critical orientation is literary, informed by the history of the book and the novel in particular. Overall, in seeking to specify my disciplinary motives,

I follow Andrew Franta, who, in his 2019 study of literary uses of disorder, acknowledges a debt to theorists of the novel who position the genre as "a vehicle for thinking about how the social world resists attempts to explain or comprehend it" (4). Reconfiguring this idea for the present volume suggests that authors use illness to show how the body and its suffering both resist and demand explanation.

Other scholars have covered some aspects of illness in Canadian literature in greater depth, including in 2019 and 2021 special issues of the journals *Studies in Canadian Literature* and *Canadian Literature* that treat themes of care and pandemics, respectively (see Hétu; Kim). Amelia DeFalco's *Imagining Care* (2018) considers caregiving in the work of several Canadian authors, including a discussion of nurses in Alice Munro's work (111–26). Marlene Goldman's *Forgotten* (2017) examines dementia in Canadian literature. Shane Neilson's theoretical 2023 study builds from the notion that healthcare is core to Canadian national identity (9) and looks to this country's literature for an origin story of its socialized healthcare. Suggesting that Canada's literature reflects the culture of care that led to its development of a single-payer system, Neilson argues "that socialized medicine came to fruition in Canada because of our collective myths and beliefs (captured in CanLit)" (21). Noting the proliferation of illness stories in Quebec literature after 1940, Julie Robert contends in *Curative Illnesses* (2016) that "the sick character's body becomes a figure for the sick nation" (5) and that illness narratives respond to anxieties regarding national change (14). In contrast to these studies, my goal is to offer an index to illness in significant works of Canadian narrative, rather than trying to suggest that gathering them together as such reveals anything in particular about our national culture, or that they explain why Canadians have, for the last few decades at least, seen fit to fund public healthcare.

Early on, a key angle of interest in this volume for me was admittedly the sense that the provision of universal healthcare was an essential feature of Canadian identity, and so a study of how this country's literature treated illness might bring us to a place of better national understanding. Yet pursuing this approach would invite the same objections leveled at the thematic criticism of the 1970s, which read Canada's literature for revelations of its overarching culture, most famously in Northrop Frye's notion of the "garrison mentality," and Margaret Atwood's claim that Canadian authors focus on survival in the wilderness above all. Over the subsequent two decades, critics rebelled against the reductionism and oversimplifications of this impulse to draw out representative themes in Canadian literature as a way of diagnosing national character (Brown). More recent calls ask critics to turn outward to the contexts that permit the emergence of literary texts, with an attendant interest in shifting the historically national organization of English studies away from an implicit focus on the nation-state (Kamboureli).

The notion of Canadian healthcare, however, does imply a national presence. To invoke Benedict Anderson's famous concept of how citizens imagine their nations into being, this presence could be said to coalesce in the minds of Canadians through their engagements with public care. Yet many histories complicate celebratory views of the healthcare system as a recognizably positive symbol of Canadian national identity. As I discuss at greater length in the fifth chapter, the idea of illness in Canada must also be understood in relation to the ongoing colonial decimation of Indigenous populations and Indigenous experiences of hospitals as carceral extensions of the residential school system. Furthermore, because the administration of health infrastructure is provincial, in practice the meaning of this system is not wholly unified under the banner of the nation, and indeed while there is evidence that English Canadians associate healthcare with a positive vision of this country, the relation is not as simple in Quebec (Dufresne et al.). Likewise, with increasing privatization across Canada, the idea that funding public healthcare is core to Canadian values and identity can't be assumed and risks becoming honoured in the breach.

As a result of all these complexities, rather than interjecting in discussions of Canadian nationalism or arguing that these stories reflect cultural support for public healthcare, my primary goal has been to observe how each book under consideration uses illness to achieve specific narrative ends. In this sense I hope that this volume is particularizing rather than universalizing, since, of course, though disease can sicken whole populations, illness looks different in each body and book.

My approach to choosing works to address here has been both broad and necessarily limited. I have taken a fairly wide perspective on narrative prose, including some nonfiction works as well as books written for younger readers. Avenues that I have not comprehensively addressed but that offer scope for further exploration include books that treat encounters in hospitals, such as *Reproduction* (2018), by Ian Williams, and M.G. Vassanji's *No New Land* (1997), popular writing by doctors beyond the work of Vincent Lam, such as Canada's most famous poem, "In Flanders Fields" (1919), by physician John McCrae, and the bestselling accounts of humanitarian medical work in international conflict zones by doctors James Orbinski (2009) and James Maskalyk (*Life on the Ground Floor*; *Six Months in Sudan*). I do not discuss the novelist Rohinton Mistry at length but he often frames postcolonial experience as a physical ailment, as seen for example in his story "Squatter" in *Tales from Firozsha Baag* (1987). In Mistry's story, a Parsi immigrant bases his sense of belonging in Canada on whether he can learn the custom of using a toilet in a seated rather than squatting position, finding in the end that life in Toronto "was just a pain in the posterior" (178). Derek Ettensohn argues that Mistry's many depictions of physical affliction throughout his writing, including disability in *Such a Long Journey* (1991) and *A Fine Balance* (1995), and Parkinson's disease in *Family Matters* (2002), illuminate the "vulnerable aesthetic" that drives his work. Another context that exceeds the focus of the book involves the cultural history of blood in Canada. As the novelist Lawrence Hill explains in his published Massey Lectures, *Blood: The Stuff of Life* (2013), blood in Canadian public consciousness has been impacted by the legacy of the "tainted blood" scandal, which spread fatal HIV and hepatitis C infections to thousands of recipients of transfusions in the 1980s (107–15). This episode, which does not appear in any of the many subsequent works I write about here, provides another example of how significant historical suffering does not necessarily receive equivalent fictional treatment.

I include texts by Indigenous authors not because they are themselves easily classified as "Canadian," but because the idea of Canadian literature cannot be understood without heeding rather than omitting Indigenous voices. Acknowledging the racist colonial history that defines this country and its culture requires spotlighting the writing of those best positioned to articulate its harms. As the final report of the Truth and Reconciliation Commission of Canada points out, "Reconciliation is not an Aboriginal problem; it is a Canadian one" (vi): contemplating the literature of this country means regarding the colonial violence on which this state was built, the enduring sickness in its foundation. Indigenous writers also depict this nation's inequitable healthcare system, and they are celebrated by Canadian awards, media outlets, and readers across the country. Indigenous authors publishing in this country do not all identify as Canadian, but reading their work is integral to understanding this country and its literary culture.

Indigenous notions of healing also open important interpretive avenues for reading the works discussed here. The Western medical model imagines that sickness has inevitably biological causes and cures, with the idea of "medicine" representing something to be consumed (see Duffin 94–98). Indigenous knowledge frameworks in contrast open a wider view of the concept of medicine and the trajectories that lead into and out of suffering, with story itself often a crucial factor, as Jo-Ann Episkenew (Métis) explains (13–14). This potential for healing through narrative should be kept in mind when encountering all the works discussed here, by Indigenous and non-Indigenous authors alike. As much as writers use illness for literary goals, they and their readers may also use stories for therapeutic ends.

In abiding by the structuring and thematic guidelines I have outlined, my selections lean towards newer, twenty-first century literature. This preference may reflect an eagerness to cast fresh eyes on fresh work, but also a curiosity about how literature reflects and responds to the fraught contemporary moment, beset as it is by so many social ills that impact health, including the underreported toxic drug crisis, institutionalized racism, and crumbling housing, medical, and climate systems. We are also at a moment when, after decades of exhortations to combat stigma of all kinds through authentic disclosure, sickness is a rising target of obfuscation. Though this reticence is partly due to a deference to privacy, in media reports people now regularly die of "health issues," an absurd formulation, given that death is the most decisive health issue of all. This phrase sweeps illness under the carpet of vague imprecision. Such unnaming looks to mask suffering, to hide—and hide from—its fearful threat. Part of my goal in this book is to counter such evasions by exposing the unflinching gaze authors cast on illness.

These chapters offer in-depth readings of key texts with reference to relevant contexts and concepts in literary theory, such as postmodernism, historical fiction, and autobiography, to assist students and teachers of literature and healthcare workers hoping for story-based considerations of their craft. My intention is to help instructors tasked with prepping classes on the fly with too little time, and medical practitioners, curious to learn more about these books, but without the apparatus of literary training to back them—and also with less time to read widely than they might like. To keep this work legible to people working across disciplines, I have tried to make my language as accessible as possible, avoiding footnotes and buzzwords that may lack meaning for many readers without, I hope, oversimplifying my topic.

I have taken the opportunity of writing this textbook as an extension of the craft of bookselling, which I have written about elsewhere ("Whims"). This reflective practice entails suggesting books to readers based on their own stated desires, and part of my goal in this work is to recommend books to you. Every work I have written about here is worth reading—for its own sake, but in some instances more especially for people with particular motivations. For example, for the social worker at Toronto's SickKids hospital, wondering how a child's devastating illness impacts the mental health of her siblings, please look to Julie Johnston's *Hero of Lesser Causes*. For a nurse taking on his first remote assignment and looking for books about illness in the vastness of the Canadian landscape, I recommend devoting some winter evenings to *Roughing it in the Bush*, *Station Eleven*, and *The Marrow Thieves*, whose conjunctions reward scrutiny. For the public health worker seeking literary context for opioid addiction, I suggest *On the Ravine* and *The English Patient*, whose distinct accounts of opiate dependency and the administration of drugs should be put into conversation. To the practitioner looking for stories to help colleagues and students reflect on how hospitals can feel hostile to Indigenous patients and healthcare workers, I recommend Michelle Good's *Five Little Indians*. These books have power to soothe the soul, as people like to say about reading, but also, or more so, to illuminate the soul—and its suffering.

Any work of selection such as what has gone into gathering the books that I address here is of course driven by the collector's taste. Mine runs toward thrilling reads, fresh voices, and historically significant or celebrated impact among readers, as measured by conversations, sales, and sometimes awards. I look to be swept away by stories and wish to introduce you to books whose significance and recognition has grown from how they leverage the full scope and might of narrative technique. The assessments driving my choices are necessarily subjective and open to critique, but I have done my best to gather a meaningful assembly of enlivening Canadian books for you to consider in relation to illness. Let's begin.

Works Cited

Anderson, Benedict. *Imagined Communities: Reflections on the Origin and Spread of Nationalism*. 1983. Verso Books, 2006.

Atwood, Margaret. *Survival: A Thematic Guide to Canadian Literature*. Anansi, 1972.

Barrows, Howard S., and Robyn M. Tamblyn. *Problem-Based Learning: An Approach to Medical Education*. Springer, 1980.

Bleakley, Alan, and Shane Neilson, editors. *Routledge Handbook of Medicine and Poetry*. Routledge, 2024.

Brown, Russell Morton. "The Practice and Theory of Canadian Thematic Criticism: A Reconsideration." *University of Toronto Quarterly*, vol. 70, no. 2, 2001, pp. 653–89.

Charon, Rita. *Narrative Medicine: Honoring the Stories of Illness*. Oxford UP, 2006.

Crawford, Paul, et al., editors. *The Routledge Companion to Health Humanities*. Routledge, 2023.

DeFalco, Amelia. *Imagining Care*. U of Toronto P, 2018.

Diedrich, Lisa. *Treatments: Language, Politics, and the Culture of Illness*. U of Minnesota P, 2007.

Duffin, Jacalyn. *History of Medicine: A Scandalously Short Introduction*. 3rd ed., U of Toronto P, 2021.

Dufresne, Yannick, et al. "The True North Strong and Free Healthcare? Nationalism and Attitudes towards Private Healthcare Options in Canada." *Canadian Journal of Political Science*, vol. 47, no. 3, Sept. 2014, pp. 569–95.

Episkenew, Jo-Ann. *Taking Back Our Spirits: Indigenous Literature, Public Policy, and Healing*. U of Manitoba P, 2009.

Ettensohn, Derek. "Rohinton Mistry's Vulnerable Aesthetic: Health, Illness, and the Body in *Such a Long Journey*." *Modern Fiction Studies*, vol. 67, no. 3, Sept. 2021, pp. 568–88.

Fifield, Peter. *Modernism and Physical Illness: Sick Books*. Oxford UP, 2020.

Frank, Arthur W. *The Wounded Storyteller*. U of Chicago P, 1995.

Franta, Andrew. *Systems Failure: The Uses of Disorder in English Literature*. Johns Hopkins UP, 2019.

Frye, Northrop. *The Bush Garden: Essays on the Canadian Imagination*. Anansi, 1971.

Goldman, Marlene. *Forgotten: Narratives of Age-Related Dementia and Alzheimer's Disease in Canada*. McGill-Queen's, 2017.

Hawkins, Anne Hunsaker. *Reconstructing Illness: Studies in Pathography*. Purdue UP, 1993.

Hétu, Dominique. "Introduction: Models of Care and Women's Writing." *Studies in Canadian Literature*, vol. 44, Dec. 2019, pp. 143–61.

Hill, Lawrence. *Blood: The Stuff of Life*. House of Anansi, 2013.

Hingston, Kylee-Anne. *Articulating Bodies: The Narrative Form of Disability and Illness in Victorian Fiction*. Oxford UP, 2019.

Hunter, Kathryn Montgomery. *Doctors' Stories: The Narrative Structure of Medical Knowledge*. Princeton UP, 1991.

Jurecic, Ann. *Illness as Narrative*. U of Pittsburgh P, 2012.

Jutel, Annemarie Goldstein. *Diagnosis: Truths and Tales*. U of Toronto P, 2019.

Kamboureli, Smaro. "Shifting the Ground of a Discipline: Emergence and Canadian Literary Studies in English." *Shifting the Ground of Canadian Literary Studies*, edited by Smaro Kamboureli and Robert Zacharias, Wilfrid Laurier UP, 2013, pp. 1–36.

Kim, Christine. "The Cultural Politics of Pandemics Representations." *Canadian Literature*, no. 245, Sept. 2021, pp. 5–12.

Kleinman, Arthur. *The Illness Narratives: Suffering, Healing, and the Human Condition*. 1988. Basic Books, 2020.

Krienke, Hosanna. *Convalescence in the Nineteenth-Century Novel: The Afterlife of Victorian Illness*. Cambridge UP, 2021.

Lucius-Hoene, Gabriele, et al., editors. *Illness Narratives in Practice: Potentials and Challenges of Using Narratives in Health-Related Contexts*. Oxford UP, 2018.

Maskalyk, James. *Life on the Ground Floor*. Doubleday Canada, 2017.

Maskalyk, James. *Six Months in Sudan: A Young Doctor in a War-Torn Village*. Random House Publishing Group, 2009.

McCrae, John. "In Flanders Fields." *In Flanders Fields and Other Poems*, Briggs, 1919.

Mistry, Rohinton. "Squatter." *Tales from Firozsha Baag*. 1987, McClelland & Stewart, 2000.

Moss, Laura. "'A Science of Uncertainty': Bioethics, Narrative Competence, and Turning to the 'What if' of Fiction." *Studies in Canadian Literature*, vol. 40, no. 2, June 2015, pp. 5–24.

Neilson, Shane. *Canadian Literature and Medicine: Carelanding*. Routledge, 2023.

Orbinski, James. *An Imperfect Offering: Humanitarian Action in the Twenty-First Century*. Doubleday, 2009.

Robert, Julie. *Curative Illnesses: Medico-National Allegory in Québécois Fiction*. McGill-Queen's, 2016.

Robertson, Colin, et al., editors. *Storytelling in Medicine: How Narrative Can Improve Practice*. 2016. 2nd ed., CRC, 2024.

Sontag, Susan. *AIDS and Its Metaphors*. Farrar, Straus and Giroux, 1989.

Sontag Susan. *Illness as Metaphor*. Farrar, Straus and Giroux, 1978.

Statistics Canada. *Leading Causes of Death, Total Population, by Age Group*. Government of Canada, 27 Nov. 2023, www150.statcan.gc.ca/t1/tbl1/en/tv.action?pid=1310039401.

Truth and Reconciliation Commission of Canada. *Honouring the Truth, Reconciling for the Future: Summary of the Final Report of the Truth and Reconciliation Commission of Canada*. Truth and Reconciliation Commission of Canada, 2015.
Vassanji, M. G. *No New Land*. McClelland & Stewart, 1997.
Vendler, Helen. *Last Looks, Last Books: Stevens, Plath, Lowell, Bishop, Merrill*. Princeton UP, 2010.
Williams, Ian. *Reproduction*. Vintage Canada, 2019.
Wolfe, Jessica Duffin. "Pandemic: Old Stories of a New Virus." *Literary Review of Canada*, vol. 28, no. 3, Apr. 2020, pp. 7–11.
Wolfe, Jessica Duffin. "Whims and Longings: In the Vicinity of That Folio." *Literary Review of Canada*, vol. 30, no. 8, Oct. 2022, pp. 23–29.
Woods, Angela. "The Limits of Narrative: Provocations for the Medical Humanities." *Medical Humanities*, vol. 37, no. 2, Dec. 2011, pp. 73–78.
Woolf, Virginia. "On Being Ill." *Selected Essays*, edited by David Bradshaw, Oxford UP, 2008, pp. 101–11.

1

PREVAILING DISORDER

Epidemics and Infectious Diseases

This chapter considers literary treatments of major epidemic diseases in Canada over the last two centuries. An epidemic illness is one that spreads in a particular region (Hammond 5). Such infectious outbreaks have had significant impacts on Canadian history, particularly through their contribution to the colonial devastation of Indigenous populations (see Daschuk; Piper). Rather than charting the full scope of historical contagion in Canada or tracing the development of Canadian narrative in general, this chapter follows the history of how major epidemic illnesses appear through the windows of celebrated narrative works.

The order of texts under discussion follows the historical chronology of the major outbreaks they portray. Starting with Susanna Moodie's 1852 chronicle of nineteenth-century cholera, malaria, and scarlet fever, I next consider Lucy Maud Montgomery's depictions of early twentieth-century tuberculosis, typhoid fever, and measles. Two works of historical fiction published two years apart, Alice Munro's "Carried Away" (1994) and Julie Johnston's *Hero of Lesser Causes* (1992), portray Ontarian struggles with the 1919 influenza pandemic and polio in the 1940s, respectively. Indigenous authors Tomson Highway (Cree) and Gregory Scofield (Métis) offer contemporaneous portrayals of the HIV/AIDS epidemic in the 1990s, with an awareness of how that outbreak echoed the impacts of colonial diseases among earlier generations. Vincent Lam's depiction of the 2003 SARS epidemic and its memorialization in Emily St. John Mandel's bestselling speculative pandemic novel bring this literary history of contagious illnesses in Canada into the twenty-first century.

DOI: 10.4324/9781003340119-2

In choosing works for this chapter I sought to illustrate the presence of historical epidemics in noteworthy narrative works. Jumping from early twentieth-century literature to historical fiction from the 1990s is not meant to imply that no books published during the intervening decades portray any illness, and indeed such texts appear in subsequent chapters. Rather my goal is to trace literary appearances of historical epidemics according to their own chronology.

As we shall see, from community outbreaks to global pandemics, contagious illnesses offer narrative opportunities to consider the lives of individuals within groups. By putting everyone at risk, outbreaks let authors weigh the value of life itself, both in the individual and collective, while the common cause of the people of a country can become visible in the suffering that they share and spread. Even as the course of illness in the body presents a story with a beginning, rising conflict, and denouement, this storyline parallels the impact of contagion on a population, from infection, to the spread of damage, to final outcome. This population-level impact, which starts in the spread of disease from one individual to another, mirrors acts of communication and social relations, and the works discussed here scrutinize how illness inflects relationships. Often the sign of a contagious infection, fever in these books can let authors indulge in indeterminacy: as temperatures rise, realist precision fades.

As infection circulates among populations, sickness puts people on the move, either to escape contagion, to visit loved ones, or to find new homes after their companions have died. The books discussed in this chapter show that even as it ends lives, illness starts stories.

Cholera, Malaria, and Scarlet Fever: Susanna Moodie's *Roughing It in the Bush* (1852)

One of the earliest works classed as Canadian literature, Susanna Moodie's *Roughing It in the Bush* (1852) begins with immigrants landing in Quebec during a cholera epidemic that troubles every port down the St. Lawrence River (21). Illness besets whatever land the settlers might touch after two months at sea, and Canada itself is a "plague-stricken spot" (50) that comes into being as a scene of contagion.

Colonial settlement in Canada transpired in tandem with decimating outbreaks of smallpox and other diseases among Indigenous populations (see Piper), but new arrivals also faced an onslaught of contagion spurred partly by their own increased international mobility. Two years after Moodie's book appeared, an English doctor would demonstrate the waterborne origins of cholera by mapping an outbreak to contacts with the now-famous Broad Street pump (Duffin, *History* 178), but in Moodie's telling, the air is "rank with pestilence" (50) and cholera is liable to jump from any number of sources, such as apples or oysters (57). Shane Nielson addresses this moment in epistemological history in his consideration of Moodie's book through the lens of public health. The first official agents the immigrants encounter are "health-officers," sent to detect and isolate sick arrivals (40–41), and "who talked much and ominously of the prevailing disorder" (41). Both immigration and epidemics throw characters into encounters with authority. On shore the scene is one of broken social relations, as those who are not ill carouse and steal with impunity (29). According to a soldier, "The healthy actually run the risk of taking cholera by robbing the sick" (31). The captain's foreboding that he would not escape death by cholera a third time after encountering it twice previously abroad mirrors Moodie's own enumeration of meetings with the illness in England and Scotland (50). International travel in this work entails a constant hopscotch around contagion.

In Moodie's telling, many significant choices of how to travel and encounter new territories are driven by illness, either in efforts to escape quarantine requirements or elude contagion (56). One immigrant family's plight strikes Moodie as most pitiable: paid by a wealthy benefactor to investigate opportunities in Canada, all was nevertheless lost, for "Their only son, a fine lad of fourteen, had died that day of the cholera, and all their hopes for the future were buried in his grave" (60). Moodie makes the dread of a broad contagion personal through the story of an individual loss. She can't explore Montreal as "The cholera was at its height" (50), while Quebec is a "plague-stricken city" (47), where "the almost ceaseless tolling of bells proclaimed a mournful tale of woe and death" (39). Officials inspecting the ship dissuade passengers from landing by describing "the frightful ravages of the cholera" on shore (51), telling them that "It will be a miracle if you escape," as "Hundreds of emigrants die daily" (51). One man, desperate to revel on land after weeks at sea, leaves his wife in boundless distress when he misses the boat: "During the reign of the cholera," Moodie writes of this scene, "what at another time would have appeared but a trifling incident, was now invested with doubt and terror" (46). If Moodie documents an early collective sensibility among this new community, it is forged in mass contagion.

Cholera is not the only illness bedevilling the settlers. Malaria, then called "ague" (Duffin, *History* 202), also features as an endemic and often-decisive obstruction. The settler Tom Wilson recounts contracting ague as a result of fatigue, resolving to leave Canada, but he is forced to stay until he recovers (82). While cholera and malaria haunt the adult settlers, children are also beset by illness. A son's malady causes Moodie to reluctantly incur a debt to a neighbour by borrowing a candle, only to have it stolen by another neighbour's hungry cat (110–11). During Moodie's own illness while her husband is on a military tour, one of her children is taken in by a wealthier family and grows accustomed to their greater comforts (466–67): illness exposes the child to other domestic worlds and class identifications. Children themselves frequently fall ill and die in Moodie's account, as when young Phoebe, a neighbour's eldest daughter, becomes feverish, and "stood but a slight chance for her life, begging under the medical treatment of three or four old women, who all recommended different treatment and administered different nostrums" (160). Moodie tries to persuade the girl's mother to call for a doctor, but "She could not be persuaded that her daughter was really in any danger, until the doctor told her that her case was hopeless" (162). Though Moodie positions the ministrations of women as useless compared to the help of the doctor, when he does appear it is only to decree that nothing can be done.

Tragedy also inheres in Moodie's depictions of illnesses among children in Indigenous communities, despite their greater knowledge of herbal remedies. An Indigenous mother carries her dying twelve-year-old boy six miles through snow to see Moodie out of hope that she might be able to offer a cure to save him from tuberculosis. She can't, and the boy dies minutes after his mother finishes carrying him home again (288–89). Another of Moodie's tales regarding ill children concerns scarlet fever in an Indigenous community, a sickness she calls "doubly terrible to those poor creatures who don't know how to treat it" (300). This lack of knowledge of the disease contributes to its virulence as one of the main illnesses that produced genocidal impacts on Indigenous communities in the nineteenth century, when it was viewed as the worst epidemic illness of the era (Piper 25). While they lacked knowledge of remedies for scarlet fever, they have a greater knowledge of treatments in general by comparison to the settlers. Moodie describes them as "very skilful in their treatment of wounds, and many diseases. Their knowledge of medicinal qualities of their plants and herbs is very great. They make excellent poultices from the bark of the bass and the slippery elm" (301). Their use of black briony produces a "fine salve for sores" and from sumach they obtain "a good remedy for the ague," while a fungus offers a remedy for stomachache whose flavour Moodie likens to quinine (301), itself an antimalarial treatment (Duffin, *History* 202). Leanne Betasamosake Simpson (Michi Saagiig Nishnaabeg) points out the racism of Moodie's depictions of Indigenous peoples and how the text itself advances the colonial theft of Indigenous land (97–100), which readers of these scenes should keep in mind.

In an anecdote that illustrates the ongoing dream state of illness faced by the immigrants, Mr. Moodie barely remembers an old friend through the haze of his malaria (367), only to have the same visitor contract the disease

(373). With one of her children also ill, and on the brink of giving birth, Moodie hires a nurse who falls ill herself within a day (323). Moodie's entire family eventually contracts malaria and suffers with it intermittently for a year (325). "It was a melancholy season," she writes,

> one of severe mental and bodily suffering. Those who have drawn such agreeable pictures of a residence in the backwoods never dwell upon the periods of sickness, when, far from medical advice . . . you are left to languish, unattended, upon the couch of pain.
>
> (324)

What might seem the most frightful of Moodie's encounters with illness she deals with most briefly. In the winter of 1839, all five of her children contract scarlet fever, which "is so fatal to children in Canada that none of [her] neighbours dared approach the house" (436). She and a helper spend three weeks tending to the children night and day; they send for the doctor but he doesn't come (436). After this exertion, she writes, "Though I escaped the fever, mental anxiety and fatigue brought on other illness, which for nearly ten weeks rendered me perfectly helpless" (436). While Moodie names scarlet fever as the scourge afflicting her children, her own illness goes unnamed. This ambiguity may speak to the lack of nineteenth-century vocabulary for mental illness such as depression, but it may also illustrate the limits of diagnosis. "Illness" may remain simply illness alone if it conforms to no known disease category. When she at last recovers, her baby sickens and the doctor predicts that the child will die (437). Though in this instance the baby survives this also unnamed illness (436), once more a doctor is described as present only to offer a prognosis: the figure of the doctor is ineffectual but nevertheless wanted.

Moodie insists Canadians are distinguished by their care for the ill. "The Canadians are a truly charitable people," she writes. "[T]hey not only generously relieve the wants of suffering strangers cast upon their bounty, but they nurse them in sickness" (205–6). In this influential early Canadian work that presents above all a vision of colonial arrival into this country, epidemic illness represents a definitive and ever-present force. The advancement of contagion mirrors the social circulation of migrants and always suffuses their relations, their hope, and their despair.

Tuberculosis, Fevers, and Measles: Lucy Maud Montgomery's Anne and Emily Books

Lucy Maud Montgomery's idyllic vision of life in Canada, which produced the country's first international literary blockbuster, also portrays the impacts of sickness on Canadians. Contagious illnesses, from whooping cough and measles to tuberculosis and typhoid fever, offer Montgomery lenses through which to view her favourite theme, the often-overlooked preciousness of life itself.

Montgomery's novels became massive successes, and *Anne of Green Gables* (1908) alone has sold a staggering fifty million copies (Ledwell and Mitchell 3). Her books were published between 1908 and 1937, a period of intense change in Canadian society and health as immigration surged and new treatments dawned even as influenza and childhood illnesses ravaged the population. In Toronto in 1901 nearly two out of every ten infants wouldn't see their first birthday (Hallman 37). In 1921, the first year with national longevity statistics (Statistics Canada), Canadian life expectancy was just 57.1 years (Decady and Greenberg 1). Many of the innovations in scientific understanding and medical care that were to drastically increase lifespans in Canada had been discovered but not yet popularized, while access and education were unequal, and the calamity of contagion was widespread.

Many scholars have examined the effects of illness in Montgomery's life and work. Janice Fiamengo considers the author's interpretation of her depression, while Anne Stiles points out that her writing reflects notions of "mind cure" (115–54). As Melissa Prycer argues, her many depictions of tuberculosis correspond to gradual shifts in medical and social concepts of the disease. Montgomery's frequent invocations of tuberculosis, then known as "consumption" ("Consumption"), illustrate how that disease tracked Canadians and, as Katherine McCuaig explains, represented an extremely common chronic and frequently fatal malady in the late nineteenth and early twentieth centuries. While Montgomery's Emily of New Moon books were being published between 1923 and 1927, the first vaccine for tuberculosis was being tested (McCuaig 83–84), though prognoses would only reliably improve with the arrival of antibiotics and other treatments in the 1940s (197). Tuberculosis may represent the most commented on disease in Montgomery's works, but many other illnesses appear.

The author frequently uses the theme of sickness to provide significant revelations or structural elements in her fiction. Montgomery's most famous character, Anne Shirley, is known for her red braids and her orphaned state. In *Anne of Green Gables*, she explains early on that her mother, "died of fever when I was just three months old. . . . And father died four days afterwards from fever too" (56). Montgomery doesn't specify the precise variety of this fever, but fans often fill in the blanks and refer to it online as either scarlet fever or typhoid fever. This ambiguity reflects the progression of medical understanding dating back to ancient Roman sources, which, as Mitchel Hammond explains, has slowly over centuries continued to differentiate febrile ailments in tandem with advancements in science. In the late-nineteenth-century period of Anne's birth, while scarlet or typhoid fevers could have taken her parents, malaria is an equally likely deadly fever and was then often implied by references to "fever" on its own (Hammond 353–55). Anne's loss of her parents causes her to bounce between households and occasions the action of Montgomery's first novel. Though their deaths represent a convenient plot device, such losses were also common, and early mortality from contagious illnesses in this period far exceeded today's levels. The shock of this young imaginative person's arrival in the quiet and staid Cuthbert household is the central conflict of *Anne of Green Gables* and it is occasioned by illness. Indeed, it is Matthew's heart trouble that causes the Cuthberts to send for an orphan, as Irene Gammel points out in her essay on the uses of *Anne* for bibliotherapy (93), so Montgomery's plot is doubly prompted by physical malady. Here, as in Moodie's book and, as we'll see, in Emily St. John Mandel's portrayals of flight from contagion, illness causes the circulation of individuals.

Montgomery portrays in Anne an often-inadvertent capacity to both poison and cure. Her early experience caring for younger children in an earlier foster home gives her a certain medical expertise (209). Her quick thinking and use of ipecac saves her friend Diana's baby sister from whooping cough, causing the doctor to praise her abilities, saying "I never saw anything like the eyes of her when she was explaining the case to me" (209). Anne Stiles reads this episode as a critique of the medical establishment (137) and points out that Anne's administration of a cure helps rehabilitate her status in the community after being punished for inadvertently getting Diana drunk (138). In this episode, when Anne famously feeds her friend currant wine instead of a nonalcoholic raspberry cordial, Diana drinks so much she becomes "awfully sick" while Marilla contends that she "just kept that bottle for sickness" (185). The poison was just a cure administered at the wrong time. These two episodes of induced illness and cure happen because of Anne's dosing of substances that girls her age aren't supposed to know about, making her readable as a loveable drug dealer who has infiltrated the Avonlea community, or a purveyor of magic fairy food from the otherworlds she talks about so much. Anne likewise nearly feeds dinner guests sauce in which a mouse had drowned because she was distracted by imagining herself as a "frost fairy" (181). Montgomery uses the risk of Anne's delivery of strange elixirs to create dramatic incidents, while her famous "queerness" (see Pike and Robinson 8) and its excuse stem from her administration of substances that both sicken and cure.

Despite the seeming foreshadowing of professional medical ability in Anne's provision of a near-miraculous cure of the baby, two books later in *Anne of the Island* it is her love interest, Gilbert, who goes to medical school (243). The fact that plucky, clever Anne would never consider training to be a doctor reflects the sexist norms of the medical profession at the time. Indeed, the world-renowned cardiology expert Maude Abbott (1868–1840), who was born close to Anne's implied mid-1860s birthdate, was refused admission to McGill University's medical school even though she'd been the valedictorian for her undergraduate class there (Gillett). Despite the mental liberty that Anne discovers through her famous imagination, Montgomery's exceptionally bright and engaging heroine lived in a world that afforded few professional paths for women. Montgomery's work is not overtly progressive, but that sense of restriction may indeed be one of the essential points of her novels: Anne explores superlative mental horizons because others are not available to girls like her.

Montgomery's often convenient use of illness to advance her storylines is clear when, as Anne enters college in *Anne of the Island*, her school friend Ruby Gillis is "dying of galloping consumption" (78). Drawing on Katherine Byrne's discussion of tuberculosis in Victorian fiction, Lesley D. Clement argues that Montgomery's portrayal of Ruby's illness reissues gendered nineteenth-century concepts of the disease. Ruby, a highly social young woman, keeps pretending that nothing is wrong (79), and the more Anne visits her sickbed, the more she seems to deny that she is unwell (84–85). During their final visit, which proves to be Ruby's last day alive, she confesses that she is afraid to die, because she cannot imagine leaving the only world she's known (105). For Anne, the result is a realization that she does not want to be caught like Ruby, pining for petty material realities when the hereafter is at hand: "The little things of life . . . must not be the things she lived for . . . the life of heaven must be begun here on earth" (108). Once more we see Anne's precious exceptionalism on display in an episode that may leave the reader feeling more sympathy for the dying Ruby than Montgomery meant to evoke.

In a return of her parents' story in this novel, a woman living in the Bolingbroke home where Anne was born gives her a pack of letters her parents exchanged shortly before "[t]hey both died of fever" (144). Again, as in the first novel in the series, it's unclear what this fever is meant to be. Letters were all that was left in the house after Anne's parents died, the new resident says, because "The furniture was all sold to pay the doctor bills" (145). The costs of illness in this world go beyond the loss of loved ones, a reality that may seem strange to twenty-first century Canadian readers, and unremarkable to those living in places without single-payer healthcare. Later in the novel Anne's longtime "chum" Gilbert, whose marriage proposal she refused, falls sick with typhoid fever (235). Knowing he may be dying makes Anne realize she's in love with him after all (236), and once more we see illness changing Anne's perspective on her life. She receives the news that he's starting to recover from his neighbour who walks by her house on the way to visit his own sick father (237). This redoubling of illness as a cause for action and revelation recurs throughout Montgomery's work.

In the three Emily of New Moon books, Montgomery takes her most autobiographical turn, and once again illness spurs the beginning of a young girl's story. The spectre of tuberculosis is the backdrop against which the characters, especially Emily, strive to build their lives. Whereas Anne Shirley's narrative starts because of the rupture caused by the death of her parents from "fever," Emily of New Moon's story opens with the death of her father from tuberculosis, an experience that echoes the author's own loss of a parent from the same disease before she turned two years old: touching her mother's cold cheek in her coffin was Montgomery's earliest memory (Bolger 2). Emily's father's early death causes everyone around her to assume that she too will succumb to the same illness (38, 129). The possibility lets Emily imagine following him to an afterlife (35) and so escape the homesickness from which she is also suffering. As for so many of Montgomery's characters, the prospect of death by disease opens the avenue to an otherworldly perspective.

Tuberculosis is a constant threat in this novel, but its most dramatic story of illness entails Emily's dangerous bout of measles. She falls ill after an afternoon spent playing with children from Derry Pond, a community where contagion has run rampant (318). While attending her, Dr. Burnley, the father of Emily's school friend Ilse, comments that the Derry Pond children who died were "Mostly French though—the kids would be out of bed when they had no business to be and caught cold" (318). Dr. Burnley's callous and discriminatory assessment reveals that early-twentieth-century Anglophone prejudice against French Canadians was more robust than his own understanding of disease. By no means could cultural difference have so impacted the prognosis of children sick with measles, though it may be that French Canadian households in the community may have had fewer resources and been negatively impacted by what we now call the social determinants of health. After Emily herself contracts measles, a school picnic between the two communities spreads the illness widely among all the children of the region, an event Montgomery describes, rather unusually, as "a perfect orgy of measles" (328).

Emily's illness and the delirium of fever let Montgomery expose revelations that might otherwise have remained uncovered. Emily's own experience of the illness is severe and worries her family. The doctor insists that they indulge her whims and relieve any worries troubling her mind. Indeed, she seems to be fussing over a story she heard about Ilse's mother, Dr. Burney's wife, who has been missing since shortly after the birth of her daughter.

She is supposed to have run away with her cousin (258), but Emily doesn't believe she would have abandoned her baby (259), and, in her delirium, keeps muttering, "She couldn't have done it—she *couldn't* have done it" (319). Through the haze of her fever, Emily declares that she has seen Ilse's mother fall into an old well (321). She insists that it be searched, which her family obliges to keep her calm as the doctor instructed, whereupon the body of Ilse's mother is discovered at last (322–24). "There is nothing hidden that shall not be revealed," says her cousin Jimmy as the discovery in the well is about to be disclosed to the doctor (323). This citation of Christian scripture references an idea in several verses in the New Testament (*King James Version*, Matthew 10:26, Mark 4:22, Luke 8:17 and 12:2), and positions Emily's illness as causing access to revelation. This Christian clairvoyance as a result of sickness recalls Saint Hildegard of Bingen, whose spiritual visons the neurologist Oliver Sacks and others linked to migraine (see Foxhall), and whose own medical writings on illness position it as a result of original sin (Glaze 136). Emily's change of state through her fever gives her a kind of clairvoyance that foretells not the future but the past. In recovery she is left changed, with "eyes that had looked into death and read the riddle of a buried thing" (329). Montgomery makes her brush with death an explicit cause of Emily's insight.

This vignette shows Montgomery's engagement with historically accurate scourges of community health and contagious threats to children, while also affording an excuse for including what might otherwise seem like an incident beyond the frame of her usual realism. As we shall shortly see, in both her use of the idea of a fever dream to access a perspective that transgresses the established limits of the narrative world, and in her reference to a Biblical sense of revelation, this scene of Montgomery's is an unlikely precursor to Alice Munro's innovations in "Carried Away."

Though Montgomery's later novels track the impact of World War I on the lost generation, the influenza pandemic of 1919–20 does not play a role. Her life, however, was significantly marked by the epidemic. She suffered greatly when she contracted the illness, and in 1919 it claimed the life of her closest friend, Frederica Campbell MacFarlane (Lefebvre 174; Rubio 206–10). *Rilla of Ingleside* (1919), the last of the Anne novels, is dedicated to Frederica. Why Montgomery did not fictionalize influenza remains a question, but, amid such major losses, contemporary emergencies may have seemed too painful to examine closely.

Throughout Montgomery's novels, contagious illness spurs narrative and revelation, giving cause to the movements of characters, their confessions, their insights about the past, their wishes for the future, and their feelings. By putting life at stake, illness brings clarity to characters.

Influenza: Alice Munro's "Carried Away" (1994)

Later Canadian fiction returned to these early epidemics. Alice Munro's short story "Carried Away" (1994) illustrates how the early twentieth-century influenza pandemic redoubled the experiences of loss faced by Canadians who had lived through the First World War. Estimates suggest that fifty-five thousand Canadians succumbed to influenza between 1918 and 1920 (Fahrni and Jones 4), roughly ten thousand fewer than died during WWI (see Cook and Stewart): these contemporaneous calamities caused mortality on a similar scale. A work of historical fiction, a genre discussed at greater length in the next chapter, "Carried Away" is a celebrated example of how Munro often uses understatement and implication to illustrate textured and elliptical accounts of women's experiences of romantic attachment and loss over time. The July 2024 news that Munro failed to act in response to her daughter's disclosure of her husband's abuse decades earlier, and her concealment of their estrangement from interviewers (Skinner), adds context to interpretations of the moral disorder driving many of her stories, including "Carried Away."

The pandemic setting of "Carried Away" provides a context of precarious life beset by illness and death. This sense of imminent demise is repeated at the end of the story when Louisa, Munro's main character, experiences a wave of confusion related to her cardiac trouble, implying that her death may be close. The layers of loss Munro piles up from the traumas of war and flu are condensed and given exquisitely painful focus in the workplace death of Louisa's love interest, Jack Agnew. Munro contrasts the shock to the community of this single fatal accident with the greater scale of lives lost in the pandemic and World War I. The incident can be read in relation to the concerns of *An Accidental History of Canada* (2024), a collection that regards this country's history through "the small accident, the intimate catastrophe, the personal disaster that may become a matter of public interest" (Belshaw et al. 7). After Jack's workplace death, Munro's narrator observes that "The victim had fought bravely in the Great War and had only been wounded once, not seriously. Many had commented on this irony" (25). Munro's story accumulates such ironies, considering why some accidents, injuries, and illnesses, both physical and emotional, prove fatal when others don't.

This story revolves around sequences of ailments, and its last act is set in motion by a medical visit: "When Louisa went to London to see the heart specialist, in the mid-fifties, she had to take the bus. She was not supposed to drive anymore" (46). Now in her sixties, her heart is failing: "The doctor, the heart specialist, said that her heart was a little wonky and her pulse inclined to be jumpy" (46). We should interpret this brand of physical ailment as purposeful on Munro's part. No mistake that the heart is the final physical target in this story that catalogues illness and injury as well as heartache: Louisa's lifetime of heart sickness has caught up with her.

From the start of the tale, illness and health saturate the atmosphere of the characters' world and they tend to connect with each other in hospitals and libraries. Louisa, the town librarian, lives in a hotel where the guests tend to talk "a little about sickness, and a lot about the War" (3), reflecting the two main calamities of their lives. Louisa enjoys a glass of wine at the hotel bar every day for her "health" (1), a premise that serves to distract from the early twentieth-century social vilification of women drinking, either alone or in company (see Hands 41–47). Later Munro reveals that Louisa has moved on to whisky, too, diminishing her argument that her drinking is for her health (13). The core action of the story begins because an enlisted library patron starts writing to Louisa from hospital. Jack Agnew is not seriously injured in the war, but he writes that "I see worse all around me and get my mind off of all that by picturing things and wondering for instance if you are still there in the library" (2). Being paused for recovery gives him time to both recollect and dwell on his memory of the librarian, but also to write to her. Louisa, we learn in her reply, experienced a similar hiatus: "I had some sickness which put me in hospital for a long time, but I am quite well now" (4). We might suspect that her illness was tuberculosis from her reference to her time in a "sanitorium," (8), a kind of convalescent hospital set up for those suffering from tuberculosis (McCuaig 26–29), but the diagnosis is not confirmed until the end of the story (57). Louisa remarks that in the sanitorium she "had a great deal of time to read" (4). Sickness and hospitalization afford time for these characters to participate in acts of communication and engage with literature. By positioning acts of literacy, reading and writing, as possible while in care, Munro lets the hospital mirror the institution of the library, which also forms an essential social space in this story.

Time in hospital also permits illicit romance to flourish. While Jack Agnew is already engaged when he finds time to write to Louisa from the hospital (12), we learn that Louisa "had been in love once, with a doctor she had known in the sanitorium" (8). "Letters had played a part that time, too" (8), Munro writes. Mores around boundary-crossing romance may have shifted over the decades, but medical ethics have prohibited doctor–patient relationships since the development of the Hippocratic Oath in ancient Greece (Miles xiv, 139–41). Though Munro leaves the details and action of this story hidden, it lies at the core of her main character's sense of self: throughout her life, Louisa silently contends with the loss of four years of her life to the sanitorium (57), the loss of the romance, and the sense that it had soured in the end:

> Her love was returned, eventually, costing the doctor his job. There was some harsh doubt in her mind about whether he had been told to leave the sanitorium or had left of his own accord, being weary of the entanglement.
>
> (8)

This "harsh doubt" is one of the injuries the episode leaves Louisa. Now, even more than at the time this story was published, and certainly more than the era in which these events are set, we have a greater vocabulary for naming sexual violations by those in medical authority over their charges. By today's standards, with romance between doctors and patients expressly prohibited in Ontario, Louisa's involvement with her doctor could have cost him his medical licence (CPSO, *Advice* and *Boundary Violations*). The "harsh doubt," therefore, may be interpreted as Louisa's sadness over whether he continued to love her, but also, as a subtext, whether the social world that they inhabit would have been sufficiently outraged by the doctor's boundary crossing to punish him, or not.

Louisa's town is fictional, but the setting for her inappropriate medical relationship is historically accurate. Munro specifies the facility with descriptive precision: "The sanitorium was on beautiful grounds up on Hamilton Mountain, and they used to meet there along the hedged walks" (19). This historical sanitorium was founded in 1906 and operated as a dedicated tuberculosis facility until 1960, including a period in the 1950s when hundreds of Inuit patients were forcibly admitted (Grant). Louisa's residence at this particular facility, as well as the assertion that she'd taken the bus fifty-seven miles from London, Ontario to see the heart specialist (42), positions her town of "Carstairs" as an imaginary Ontario location (rather than the real Carstairs, Alberta). The contrast between the precise historical location of the hospital and the imaginary locale of Louisa's home illustrates how the publicity of medical facilities contrasts with the relative secrecy of the private lives whose details Munro relates.

Though being hospitalized in this story gives patients time to read and write, it also lets them pursue indiscretions and adulteries. While her overnight tryst with Frarey happens because "[h]is wife was in the hospital with the flu" (14), the man she eventually marries is available because his wife "had died in 1919, in the last flurry of the Spanish flu, when everyone had got over being frightened" (27). For Munro, the flu permits a Shakespearean scrambling of bodies in beds. As people are swapped in and out of hospital beds, their partners trade out new bedroom companions, an illicit reality in times of desperate pandemic conversations about hospital capacity and bed availability. Here we see Munro characteristically implying, if not fully expressing, covert aspects of human relations.

From one view, the flu provides Munro with convenient ways to orchestrate arrivals and departures of characters. From another perspective, her story offers an historically astute portrayal of what social worlds must have been like in this strange overlapping period in Canadian history, when those with both visible and invisible wounds from WWI were striving to recreate a sense of normalcy in a context troubled by a new devastation. This cognitive dissonance and the sheer scale of loss occasioned by the pandemic, which, like the Great War, claimed tens of thousands of Canadian lives, were not frequently recalled until the emergency of COVID-19 brought past events to mind again. Indeed, the coronavirus seems to have returned "Carried Away" itself to critics' minds (see Sopiarz; Darroch).

In Louisa's encounter with the travelling salesman Jim Frarey, Munro offers a portrayal of the social conditions caused by the flu that COVID-19 made familiar once more. The description of the moment—"in the early winter of 1919, when there had been a fresh outbreak of flu after the danger was supposed to be past" (14)—underscores the precarity of life in a pandemic, when moments of relative calm and feelings of safety can suddenly be shattered. Munro recounts how "They discussed the crush in the hospitals, the deaths of doctors and nurses, the unceasing drear spectacle of the funerals" (13), all images that were repeated around the world between 2020 and 2022. Their discussion of restrictions echoes arguments made during COVID lockdowns, as Frarey thinks it outrageous that churches closed: "the cowards," he complains (12). He himself "kept travelling all through the Spanish flu epidemic, though you never knew then if stores would be open for business or not" (12). Though "Few people came in, because of the flu" (17), Louisa only closes the library "when she herself was sick" (12) and had to be hospitalized. She defies public health guidelines for romantic reasons: she finds out her soldier is coming home, and "It was then that she decided to keep the library open, though the flu was raging" (16). Mark Humphries suggests that, though closure orders for public spaces may have often been forcefully issued at this time, they were not always followed (111–12). We see Munro's character weighing the risk of contagion against the desire for romantic union after the ruptures of World War I. "Even when she was sick in the hospital," Munro writes, "her only thought was that she must get back" (17). Munro thus explores a moral balance between romantic connection between two lovers and the death and illness of many strangers. For Louisa, the trade-off would be worth it, which is why she defies health restrictions. Munro's recounting of the social impacts of the flu, as well as the emotional choices that individuals make in response, places this component of her story firmly within a tradition of social and historical realism.

This realist mode is not the only register of the story, however, and illness also offers Munro a way to give it decidedly unrealistic features. The idea of illusions arising during fevers recurs throughout Munro's story. Jack Agnew writes to Louisa that he loves her because "the idea I won't ever see Carstairs again makes me think I can say anything I want. I guess it's like being sick with a fever" (10). Illness here offers a way out of the restrictions of the everyday world, in which we know (but Louisa doesn't) that he is engaged to someone else (12). Being feverish is a condition that permits one to enter the domain of the fiction writer and "say anything." When she comes upon news of Jack Agnew's return to the town, Louisa is "arranging fresh newspapers on the racks and his name jumped out at her like something in her feverish dreams" (17). Readers should be alert to this repetition of this idea of fever dreams, and, as with any interpretation of Munro, refuse to read its significance at face value. These characters, living their lives in and out of hospital and sickness, are acquainted with fever dreams as another register for reality, another form of perception. Readers should question whether illness truly frees the tongue, or permits insight, or whether it gives Munro and these characters excuses for their lapses and indiscretions.

Louisa's physically disruptive experience of seeing Agnew's name in a newspaper recurs at the end of the story, when she reads what seems to be an impossible notice of his planned appearance at a community gathering (47). Munro suggests that "Perhaps it was what she had been reading that had made her pulse jumpy" (46). Agnew's name is always appearing in texts in this librarian's world, in newspaper reports on his return (16), marriage (17) and death (28–25), on his resurrection as a union leader (47), in letters and on his library card (2), a ghostly reappearance that underscores his persistent failure to appear to her in person. This repetition of Agnew's name in print stands in contrast to the many times he does not leave a name in the library, either when borrowing books (29), or leaving a note for Louisa (18). Discovering his imminent presence gives Louisa "a faintly sickening, familiar agitation" (48). Munro leaves readers to choose whether this sense of feeling unwell derives from the prospect of seeing a dead man reborn, or whether it causes the disordered view of reality that permits such an impossible notion. While the idea of a fever dream lets Agnew imagine he can say anything, Louisa's heart ailment seems an excuse for her to perceive anything.

Munro's description of Louisa feeling faint illustrates the experience of narrative itself. As readers, we are party to the fever dream Munro creates. By the end of her encounter, Louisa is completely disoriented and seems to have missed her bus home (57). Munro describes Louisa as having "gone under a wave" that left her "with a cold sheen on her skin, a beating in her ears, a cavity in her chest, and revolt in her stomach" (56). The glitch in her perception that has caused her to see Agnew as Frarey either caused or is caused by the disorder in her body. Going under this wave parallels the experience of immersion in reading, as Miriam Marty Clark explores in her discussion of allegories of reading in this story and in this scene in particular. Munro continues, "It was anarchy she was up against—a devouring muddle. Sudden holes and impromptu tricks and radiant vanishing consolations" (56). While this passage represents the physical and mental turmoil Louisa is experiencing as she attempts to rationalize having a conversation with a long-dead man, it also describes Munro's narrative style. We can see "sudden holes and impromptu tricks" in the playful dead seriousness with which she leaves out elements that might allow this sequence to make sense, as well as the "radiant vanishing consolations" she offers readers and her characters in giving them new ways to understand their experiences. In this story, Munro creates a radiant vanishing consolation in how Agnew—killed in a workplace accident in the factory owned by Louisa's future husband, which she would come to own and profit from (52)—is reborn as a union leader, fighting every day for workers' rights (47). Robert Lecker reads the stakes of this startling turn in relation to the history of Canadian industrialism. Recalling the earlier suggestion that it was ironic for a veteran to die in an accident, Agnew's rebirth as a union leader is not so much an irony as a spectral consolation, a "what if" to help Louisa's pain go away. As readers, we are left to question the challenges and frictions in our own processes of interpretation.

Whereas the unspecified fever of Anne Shirley's parents permits her free radical trajectory through the world and the delirium of Emily of New Moon lets Montgomery push her story into the realm of the fantastic, for Munro, the fever dream is an excuse to sidestep rather than abandon realist depiction. Munro uses the idea of fever to tell what Miriam Marty Clark describes as a realist story with two divergent outcomes.

By comparing the hallucinations of storytelling and the experience of narrative to fever dreams, Munro offers a way forward for understanding the unreason of her story. Louisa's ill health gives Munro a structure for her reorganization of realism. Nothing like this should make sense, unless the scene is being focalized by someone experiencing lapses in full comprehension of the world around her due to her failing heart. And yet fiction itself shouldn't make sense either, and in this sense, we can interpret this story, which is obsessed with books and reading and spaces created by and for literature and storytelling, as digesting itself, explaining itself as one more fever dream in the history of reading.

Munro consolidates her reorganization of realist structure by ending her story with the chronological start of Louisa's time in Carstairs. The story ends with its beginning, in that in its final paragraphs Munro returns to the sequence of events that landed Louisa in the town, her arrival there at the moment the previous librarian had died (57), with her own recovery from tuberculosis still fairly recent. We can read this return as a result of Louisa's complete disorientation in time as well as place. As we find her back in Carstairs on the day of the librarian's death, we might wonder if this is also the day of Louisa's death in London. She gets the librarian's job by saying she

> had worked in Eaton's Book Department before she switched to travelling. She did not think it necessary to tell them that she had only worked there five months when she was discovered to have t.b., and that she had then spent four years in a sanitorium. The t.b. was cured, anyway, her spots were dry.
>
> *(57)*

This casual retelling of her illness mirrors a medical case history, and its placement at the end of the story serves as a reminder of how the illness itself sparked these events. Her illness is something to conceal, one of the "open secrets" of Munro's book by that title, but so is the romantic scrape she got herself into during her time as an invalid.

Munro's story is in some sense a diagnostic explanation for Louisa's life of lovesickness: though her tuberculosis was cured, her heartache was not. As in Montgomery's books, when death by illness frequently sends orphans on their way to the experiences her novels recount, Louisa's tuberculosis, and her affair with the doctor that results, is the trouble that sets the events of Munro's story in motion. The author only gestures to that earlier love story, but as readers we are left to understand it as a decisive experience in Louisa's past. The story closes with Louisa's view of the streets in Carstairs when she first arrives in spring as soon to be covered in leaves, promising that "So much that lay open now would be concealed" (58). This line reverses a citation of the biblical sentiment referenced earlier in the work of Montgomery. While the scriptural versions of this line insist that the hidden will be revealed, in this story, concealment and obfuscation form the natural motion of social worlds. We can interpret Munro's story as the leaves, concealing as well as laying open Louisa's life and her many love affairs that can't be talked about. Given its great impact on Louisa, and Munro's excision of its details from her narrative, the object of the greatest concealment is her time in the sanitorium. In this sense, the sickness at the heart of this story is both Louisa's tuberculosis and the moral disorder that would lead a doctor to pursue an affair with a patient, thereby impacting her entire future life.

Polio: Julie Johnston's *Hero of Lesser Causes* (1992)

Julie Johnston's Governor General's Award-winning children's novel about the 1940s polio epidemic in the Ottawa Valley, *Hero of Lesser Causes* (1992), traces the torment of a twelve-year-old girl in the face of her thirteen-year-old brother's paralytic illness. As he progressively loses capacities they once enjoyed together, from just lounging around the house, to swimming at the local pool where he contracted the illness, this coming-of-age story does not track a romance or education, but rather a child's discovery of helplessness in the face of another person's pain. As Keely says, "The day Patrick got sick was the last day of my childhood, as far as I was concerned" (53). The story questions how sickness does or doesn't change both the ill and their loved ones and so offers a granular view of an epidemic that ravaged many Canadian communities before the arrival of the first effective polio vaccine in 1955 (Mawdsley 460).

As a new occupational therapist in the 1960s, Johnston worked with children with physical and mental disabilities at the Ontario Hospital School (Library and Archives Canada), later renamed the Rideau Regional Centre and closed by the Ontario government in 2009 (*Closing*). Former residents won a lawsuit alleging abuse in 2013 ("Settlement"), and the next year Ontario premier Kathleen Wynn apologized for the institution's treatment of children (CTV Ottawa). Johnston would have seen first hand the impact of disability on the lives of children who were institutionalized at this time, and the distress caused to families left incapable of caring for them properly.

Johnston's story opens in the summer of 1946 (5) in "a small town in the lower Ottawa Valley" (8) during a heat wave that "continued for more than a week" (12). Keely and her brother are not allowed to go to the local pool because of "germs," but they defy their parents to escape the heat (6). In response to a question about the risk, Keely says, "you don't get germs, you get polio or something. But that's only in cities" (6). This flight from heat to a site of contagion foreshadows what are now familiar links between a warming climate and the spread of disease from animals and other sources. That Patrick has contracted the disease dawns slowly on him and those around him: at first he lacks energy (12–13), then he has a "pinched look" (18), and then he collapses, finally acknowledging, "I think I'm sick" (19). Johnston discloses his diagnosis through the community's public health response to finding the epidemic has arrived in its environs: "Channing closed its public swimming pool when it was learned that Patrick Connor had come down with a severe case of polio" (19). The community also gives their prognosis: "Everyone in town said he would die" (19), but "Patrick didn't die. He became paralyzed" (20).

The book charts Keely's own malaise as a result of her brother's illness, and shows how affliction breaks down boundaries between characters, or how thin they become when one character is harmed by another's diagnosis. Before he gets sick, Keely says, "sometimes I think I'm only here because Patrick's here, that may be without him I'm not even a person . . . I feel that if Patrick disappeared, I'd disappear too" (5). Her strong identification with Patrick causes her trouble in the face of his profound illness. "When the ache was really bad that fall," she says, "with Patrick away in the city in a hospital the size of Buckingham palace, I used to skip school at recess and say I was sick. I was sick" (20). The repetition of simple statements of illness show the intense identification between Keely and her brother. In an emotional contagion, his illness makes her ill too. Johnston stages the hope and disappointments of such chronic illness through Keely's eyes. When word arrives that he's coming home from hospital, she assumes the best, saying "I didn't know Patrick could get better all of a sudden like that" before her mother cooly replies, "He didn't" (23). The book is a tight study of the powerlessness felt by everyone in the wake of a loved one's illness and disability. Patrick foretells that for his whole life he will "be like a rag doll handed on from one nurse to the next" (61). The feeling is worse than his physical ailments, and it too is catching. Keely wants nothing more than to rouse her brother from his despondency, but becomes marked by her own sense of despair and loss of interest in her own life (144). When Patrick claims he has the right to die, saying, "It's my life," she retorts, "Maybe, but it's pretty well mixed up with mine" (144). Keely struggles to view herself as distinct from her brother. The story offers a novel example of an illness narrative as told by a person who is not sick, and who must come to terms with their own separateness from and powerlessness to change what their loved one is experiencing.

Through this tale, the aftermath of World War II offers a backdrop for Patrick's physical suffering. His nurse had cared for injured soldiers in London (46), while the nearby home for disabled veterans eventually offers him a community and location to explore an identity beyond his family. The damage of a lost veteran, suffering from amnesia, significant facial scarring, and an amputated arm, positions the harms of war as a parallel for the ravages polio wreaks on Patrick's body (80–81). Joking that he's using a wheelchair because of "An old war injury" (128) gives Patrick a way to normalize a conveyance that he at first resists. Spending time with the disabled veterans at the home gives him a social outlet, partly because "Neither of the men seemed surprised by Patrick's chair"

(119). The veterans' home also seems to be the one local destination with a ramp: as Bess Williamson explains, efforts to accommodate injuries suffered during the two World Wars advanced accessible design. Connecting a generation of amputees with those suffering from disease-caused paralysis, Johnston thus offers a neat comparison of how the physical desecrations of war prefigured those of the polio epidemic, with both causing affliction on a scale rarely seen before.

Another infectious disease, measles, also impacts the lives of these characters. Patrick befriends a shell shock victim, who in turn starts coughing with suspected measles, giving the prospect of friendship a deadly risk (96). One of Keely's friends cancels birthday plans because she has caught measles (167). Patrick's favourite nurse goes on an extended leave because she too contracts the illness (128). Her replacement, Mrs. Whinney, does not treat Patrick properly, and makes him "feel powerless" (130). "You know, for a few days last week," he says, "I thought life might almost be worth living, but it isn't. I know that now. There will always be a Mrs. Whinney out there waiting for me. I *am* powerless" (131). Measles takes his preferred companion and returns his sense of helplessness, and he says he wishes he'd gotten the measles too (131). This despair prompts his suicide attempt by swallowing too many of his pills (135). While the novel as a whole is set in motion by Patrick's polio diagnosis, if Peggy hadn't fallen ill, the unkind nurse wouldn't have arrived and made Patrick so unhappy: illness causes trouble, and contagion causes narrative.

The children are persistently weighing what might happen in real life versus their imaginations, and Patrick's insistence that "In real life you don't get happy endings" (125) leaves the book's own ending in question. The narrative ends on a note of jubilation as Patrick lifts his knee for Keely for the first time (178), but we are left to wonder how the rest of his life progresses, and whether he might spend it in an institution. Early on an unsympathetic and incompetent nurse comments that "He'd be far better off in a Home" (36). Given the documented history of abuse and neglect in such Canadian institutions during the twentieth century, this seems unlikely, and we can read Johnston's novel as a wish-fulfilling alternative history for the sorts of children she might have encountered at the Ontario Hospital School, a version of their story where they got to stay at home, with beloved siblings and family members. When Patrick attempts suicide, Keely says "He seemed to look intently at me, as if he were memorizing me" (135). Memorialization is an impulse of narrative and one way to understand storytelling, which we should keep in mind as we interpret Keely's first-person narration. The unsettling option the ending implies is that this vision of Patrick raising his knee is how Keely wants to remember him, that the book is her effort to "look intently" to memorize him and freeze his story in a version that ends on a happier note, rather than the misery and solitude suffered by many children left disabled by polio in the 1940s.

From Smallpox to HIV/AIDS: Tomson Highway's *Kiss of the Fur Queen* (1998) and Gregory Scofield's *Native Canadiana* (1996)

HIV/AIDS is another epidemic that, like smallpox a hundred years earlier, has continued the colonial decimation of Indigenous populations in Canada. Métis poet Gregory Scofield's and Cree novelist and playwright Tomson Highway's literary treatments of this illness demonstrate the complexities of its attack and damage among Indigenous communities.

Though smallpox was the primary pathogen driving contagious mortality among Indigenous communities during the early colonial period (see Daschuk), that illness has received little fictional treatment in Canada. Cree author David A. Robertson's graphic novel *Scars* (2010) stands as an interesting exception for young readers. Indigenous populations through the early twentieth century also suffered greatly with tuberculosis and influenza (see Piper), and Stó:lō author Lee Maracle's *Ravensong* (1993) explores the aftermath of an influenza epidemic and the threat of disease in a Pacific coast community (see Leggatt; Fraile-Marcos and López-Serrano). The spread of HIV from the late twentieth century on represents another contagious disease that continues to mete out disproportionate harms in Indigenous communities. Due to the centuries-long health effects of colonial violence, Indigenous populations have tended to suffer greater levels of addiction, poverty, and imprisonment, social determinants of health that predict higher HIV infection rates (Negin et al.). Canada is now the only G7 country to have a rising HIV case count (House), and the virus continues to be more prevalent in Indigenous communities than others in this country (Challacombe). While smallpox is the contagious illness most often associated with colonial harm in Canada, HIV/AIDS must also be remembered in this context.

Alongside its celebration of modern Cree culture and its devastating portrayal of abuse in a residential school, Highway's *Kiss of the Fur Queen* (1998) offers perhaps the most poignant fictional treatment of HIV/AIDS published in Canada. Highway's novel has generated a wealth of critical responses, regarding for example its portrayal of Cree narrative and healing (Braith), classical music (Krotz; Olaveson), and the Weetigo myth (Kang). Noting how Highway's novel counters the relative lack of Canadian literary representations of HIV and AIDS, Shoshannah Ganz illustrates the culture of silence that has masked the presence of this illness in Canada. Highway both plays with and critiques this secrecy.

Highway's depiction of the ravages of this disease through the story of two brothers, Gabriel and Jeremiah, transpires within an environment saturated with awareness of how epidemic illness has already devastated Indigenous communities. Their grandmother was "one among many to have succumbed to tuberculosis" (19), while a friend educates Jeremiah about the "smallpox blankets" that colonizers used as weapons of biological warfare (148). The boys, who are the two youngest of seven, "would have had ten older siblings but for TB, pneumonia, and childhood ailments" (24). Moving from tuberculosis in the early twentieth century to AIDS later shows Highway's historically precise discussion of the epidemics that impacted Indigenous populations in Canada. Highway's novel examines the inexplicability of contagious illness, even as the sickness of individual bodies becomes a key indicator and symbol of harms perpetrated against the community.

One of Highway's main concerns is finding language for pain, and throughout he frames this challenge both as a search for vocabularies in Cree or English or the Italian of musical notation that give titles to each section, but also as the struggle and refusal to tell loved ones about trauma, fear, harm, and sadness. Keeping secrets for these characters is a means of keeping going. The questioning of swapped vocabularies starts early on: the priests at the school replace Jeremiah's original name with a Catholic one that sticks through long use, despite its application by perpetrators of abuse (54). Language is fraught when even saying one's own name is a forced concession to an abuser. The boys' suffering at the hands of the priests is nightmarish (78–79). Whether or not they will tell parents about the abuse becomes a question of whether it can be assimilated into Cree. Though residential school partially steals their mother tongue from the brothers, it remains their most intimate and emotional language. On a visit home, after hearing a traditional horror story that uses the Cree word for "bad dream power" (308), Gabriel asks, "Do '*machipoowamoowin*' mean what Father Lafleur do to the boys at school?" (91). Though they steep their children in Cree mythology, the boys' parents permit no conflict with the Catholic church, and their sons never tell them what they suffered. Both sons pursue artistic careers, perhaps as an outlet for pain they cannot or will not express in words, though their concealment spreads: Gabriel at first lies to his brother about learning to dance (159), a habit of secrecy that is one legacy of his abuse. As an adult, Jeremiah hears a child use the Cree myth of a "weetigo," "a monster who eats little boys" (271), to explain his own sexual abuse: "A Weetigo ate me," the child says (271), in a devastating use of Cree to disclose the harm he has suffered and circumvent the silence and secrecy that often hides assault in this novel.

The novel charts the characters' many travels almost as a kaleidoscopic repetition with variations striating out from the prize-winning dogsled journey that opens the book (3). The boys travel to and from residential school to their northern home (48, 67, 68, 88), then to school in Winnipeg (96), and Gabriel keeps on going, travelling the world as a dancer. His departures from home to the abuse of residential school gives an origin to the international roaming that it seems makes him vulnerable to a new contagion. After getting tested for HIV, he enjoys a liaison with a stranger behind the clinic, "employing all the trickery he had acquired in Paris, Copenhagen, Sydney, Tokyo" (282). Gabriel's partner Newman takes a cruel and jealous view of him during his performance with Jeremiah: Newman

> would fool himself no longer. . . . behind the show of innocence and northern piety, what a piece of dirt, a slut, a whore, a slab of meat fucked through every orifice, from Tokyo to Toronto, from Rome to Buenos Aires.
>
> *(266)*

Here the geography of the planet is overlaid as a corollary to the expanse of Gabriel's body, with its orifices like ports of call. Newman's dour and jealous condemnation matches the geographic spread of HIV to Gabriel's sexual adventurousness, an interest in experimentation and escape that Highway associates with the legacy of his abuse. Highway thus draws a subtle moral line between the immoral cruelties of the priests and the devastation that sexual wanderlust spread in the form of HIV. If Gabriel had not been so mistreated, the book implies, he might not have sought out so many different lovers, thereby, like so many victims of the epidemic, both contracting HIV and spreading it. While Highway's novel can be read as historical fiction, documenting known tragedies from the perspective of individuals, one of its allegorical dimensions is how it thus frames the harms of a sexually transmitted disease as a metaphor for horrific sexual abuse.

The discovery of Gabriel's illness dawns slowly. He remarks on a spot, wondering, "What's this? The blemish on his neck still there? After two weeks?" (275) He is persistently ill: "Gabriel had had the flu twice this year, so this might be the third, but was anyone immune at this time of the year?" (275) Gabriel's partner chastises him, saying, "If you didn't do so much running around, you wouldn't get sick so often" (274). Newman's jealous irritation at Gabriel's adventurousness does inadvertently touch on an aspect of the contagion at hand, the circulation that has spread the disease. At the testing clinic full of young men, Gabriel tries to imagine himself back on the lake where he grew up, "Except that Mistik Lake was filled not with water but with fresh human blood" (281). As Gabriel gets sicker, despite the doctor's advice, he doesn't stop performing, smoking, drinking, or having transactional sex (294–95). Soon the illness is just another feature to hide with stage makeup before his performances: "When he arrived at that now familiar blemish on the right side of his neck, he brushed it over with the honey-beige base until the purplish red could pass for a hickey" (283). Though admitting he is sick takes Gabriel time, the illness itself is soon just something to cover up.

Gabriel's illness gives the concealment within his family another focus. When he finds out he is HIV positive right before a performance (284), he whispers to his lover, "please don't . . . tell Jeremiah" (285). When his brother asks what pills he's taking, he says, "Vitamins. My . . . cold feels like it's . . . coming back" (293). The habit of not telling their parents about their abuse becomes a practice of not talking about the disease: in both cases, sickness lies at the heart of the silence. As Gabriel's illness progresses, Latin medical vocabularies for his medication and ailments become another verbal register throwing up a barrier to disclosing his suffering to his mother:

> How to explain pentamidine, let alone *Pneumocystis carinii*, that rare pneumonia one got only when something had kicked the hell out of one's natural immunities? How to explain the virus in his bloodstream, let alone how he had come by it?
>
> *(292–93)*

The words he now lives with seem inexplicable, and their impenetrability matches his reluctance to disclose the personal history that put him in the path of HIV. The brothers argue about whether and what to tell their mother, and Gabriel doesn't want to say anything at all: "How do you say AIDS in Cree, huh? Tell me, what's the word for HIV?" he demands (296). The two kinds of language, the ancient world of Cree and the medical acronym for a postmodern epidemic, seem impermeable, perpetuating the by-now automatic secrecy between the family members.

The struggle for language and disclosure is part of Highway's exploration of responsibilities shared between children and adults. When she sees her son on his deathbed at last, the boys' mother elides the struggle for words with a single Cree utterance: "*Nigoosis, nigoosis, nigoosis*," she repeats (300), the Cree word for "my son" (309). Finding language in Cree for HIV is unnecessary when kinship can still be declared. Harkening back to an early childhood moment when he saved Gabriel from a herd of caribou (45–47), Jeremiah castigates himself for not also protecting Gabriel the adult. His brother tries to reassure him: "I'm not a child any more, Jeremiah. Haven't been for a long time. . . . What I did, I did on my own" (300). Highway thus raises questions of children and responsibility, of whether children can be responsible for each other, of what kind of burdens children are on each other, and the harm done to them by giving them adult concerns. As Gabriel suffers on his deathbed with nightmares of the Weetigo bearing a crucifix toward him, his mother arrives with a crucifix of her own: she "placed the rosary on Gabriel's chest, the naked, silver Jesus glinting in the candle light, writhing in pain" (300). Present and dangling against the children's faces during the rapes they suffer (57, 78), the crucifix—the emblem of Christ's own trajectory from blessed infant to tortured adult—becomes a symbol of the brothers' abuse as children and their pain as grown men, in their torment as survivors and in the ravages of AIDS.

The novel closes with a medical allegory for institutional and systemic racism, as the effort to burn sweetgrass for Gabriel on his deathbed sets off the smoke detectors at the hospital (304). When questioned, Jeremiah tries to explain the ritual to a nurse, saying it's "like incense for Catholics" (304), once more showing the inescapability of their abusers' culture when trying to explain their own. Their mother, still devoted to Catholicism, tries to bring a priest, while the fire chief also arrives (305), as Highway plays with the question of whose authorities attend to death. The fire chief insists the sweetgrass be extinguished, saying, "Sir, unless the smoke detector inside that room is stopped, the whole hospital has to be evacuated" (305). This threat to evacuate the entire hospital because of one patient burning sweetgrass offers an allegory of the impact of institutional racism. An individual's effort to practise cultural rituals that should be innocuous within the broad scale of the nation or hospital is targeted as a source of trouble or contagion that could impact the whole, and that is persecuted as a result. The medical setting gives Highway a tight frame that could be extrapolated even beyond the hospital, to the institution of the country itself.

As an important poetic corollary to Highway's novel, Gregory Scofield's *Native Canadiana: Songs from the Urban Rez* (1996) offers another Indigenous author's perspective on the AIDS epidemic. In noting how Scofield's elegiac poems regarding the epidemic and its thefts avoid naming HIV/AIDS directly, Sara Jamieson connects this verbal reticence to stigma (54), a social obstruction with which Highway also contends. In Scofield's poem "Queenie," the illness of the speaker's dead lover makes them think "I too would be a goner" (68), showing the risk of mortality AIDS gave love. In "Another Street Kid Just Died" (103), the speaker mourns a queer Indigenous youth who cared for his community. They are left to wonder "if he jumped or was pushed/out the hotel window downtown" because, the speaker says, "Last week around/the office I found out he had the plague" (103). The injustice and tragedy of AIDS reflects the terrible daily threats to Indigenous and queer youth, who experience violence at among the highest levels in Canada (Heidinger). Scofield dedicates "The Owls in the City" to "my *Âyahkwêw* relations," using the Cree word for the dual-gendered concept of "Two-Spirited" people (72). This term can refer to a broad range of sexual preference as well as fluid gender identity and refers to a community of people who were severely afflicted by the initial spread of HIV. In Scofield's poem, these relations are "all sick or dead/or just about" (71). The speaker feels the strangeness of having been spared their sexual interest, and therefore their illness, too: "Because I screamed and hollered/they kept out of my pants" (71). The speaker here is reminiscing about a time "back in the '80s/before the plague really hit," saying, with the Cree word for "people," "Today it's worse—/our *iyiniwak* are dropping/like rotten chokecherries/in back alleys or hospitals" (72). The speaker here compares the tidal losses of the epidemic to a seasonal shedding of fruit from trees, a sense of living abundance wasted. This juxtaposition of the hiddenness of the back alley with what Foucault describes as the hospital's scene of observation (134–36) underscores how neither promises safety in the context of a prejudiced society and a merciless illness. "Even owls have migrated to the city," the speaker laments, "hooting their miserable death chant" (172). The idea of owls in the city gives words to the speaker's sense of displacement and loss in the face of AIDS: the strangeness of owls in the city serves as a metaphor for the weird departures of those who shouldn't have left.

SARS and the Age of the Coronavirus: Vincent Lam's "Contact Tracing" (2005)

Well before COVID-19 began gathering force for its global onslaught, the world encountered another coronavirus that, in retrospect, foreshadowed the havoc its cousin would unleash, and proved to have been a lucky near miss by comparison. Nearly eight hundred people died in the outbreak of a coronavirus called SARS in 2003 (WHO), a number that has since been dwarfed by the more than seven million confirmed COVID-19 deaths (WHO Health Emergencies), but that at the time represented a terrifying loss. What is not always remembered is that while roughly one percent of documented Canadian cases of COVID-19 prove fatal ("Mortality"), SARS cut down an estimated ten percent of the people it infected: it was a far more deadly virus (Pormohammad et al.). Like COVID-19, SARS was initially viewed by the international community as primarily a problem for China, leading to anti-Asian racism. Yet Canada was one of the most affected countries, with Toronto and Vancouver significantly impacted (Duffin, "Introduction" 1–2), highlighting the thick international ties of this country's large cities. Many of the features of SARS, the quick jump from animals to humans (Hammond 464), the instant global contagion due to the broad dispersal of social networks and the ease of air travel, proved to be rehearsals for the eventual massive spread of COVID-19.

Physician and author Vincent Lam's short story about doctors working in a hospital during the 2003 SARS epidemic serves as an important memorial of that time in Canadian history. Published in *Bloodletting and Miraculous Cures* (2005), "Contact Tracing" presents fiction itself as a kind of contact tracing, explaining why some characters connect with others, and what the trajectories of those relationships are, and what contagion or strife is caused or avoided as a result. The action of the story is interspersed with reports and medical records that provide another perspective on the events. The uncertainty of an uncontained pathogen disrupts easy authority and prognosis and troubles history, raising the question of whether anyone will survive to witness what transpires and tell the story afterward. Laura Moss points out that Lam's interest in uncertainty can be connected to William Osler, whose suggestion that "medicine is a science of uncertainty and an art of probability" begins *Bloodletting and Miraculous Cures* as an epigraph, and whose impact on twentieth-century medical pedagogy through the demand that doctors attend to the uncertain is being felt once more in the rise of narrative medicine and its use in medical training.

Bloodletting and Miraculous Cures is a series of stories connected by their recurring characters, whom we will meet again in *On the Ravine* (2023). In "Contact Tracing," Lam focalizes the characters' social intersections as sources of both friendship and contagion. Readers are treated to Delores's history because she's assigned as Fitz's nurse (281), and we get his backstory with Ming because of their prior contact and his proximity to her husband Chen (279). The illness spreads between people as though they are themselves regions, bringing with it "panic spreading like flight trajectories between cities" (287). Fitz, who works as a doctor on planes, contracts and spreads SARS because he was on a medical team tending to a sick patient on a transfer from Shenzhen to Vancouver. "Now the patient was dead," Lam writes, "which was also not outside routine, but what was new was that they were sick, they had made others sick, and the whole world was now holding its breath while learning this new word, SARS" (275). Illness occasions new vocabularies, while the spread of a new pathogen changes the impact of illness and the roles and risks of doctors. Facing his guilt over being an agent of the spread, Fitz laments to Chen that "I gave you this SARS thing," to which his friend retorts, "It's an infection. It's not you" (279). The deeply personal experience of illness and spread leads patients to identify with the pathogen. Chen and Fitz's visibility to each other is unlike most people's experience in isolation, allowing them to chat, and reminisce about a colleague who died of cancer (283–86), an ironic introduction of another illness that, in contrast to SARS, is not contagious. SARS, like any infectious disease, both brings people too close to each other, by letting them infect each other, and separates them more than they'd like.

Lam also considers the obstruction posed by SARS to personal connection through the barrier of the medical mask. As the nurses are asked who will resign or join the lottery for SARS-ward assignment, "they looked at their colleagues, but because of the masks could not tell whether the glances were farewell smiles, gazes of consolation, or eyes met as a warning" (282). Fitz is so concerned about spreading the illness that he requests a Do Not Resuscitate designation to ensure none of his colleagues intubate him, since the procedure tends to spread the virus (297–98). Chen, already having been infected, brings Lam's exploration of the social proximities and barriers caused by contagion to a peak by breaking through a glass wall to revive Fitz when he collapses (305). This story, which uses the concept of contact tracing to circle how the pathogen disrupts social connection, closes by pointing out that in Hong Kong there is community spread (305), obviating the benefit of storytelling to map contacts. Fiction itself becomes unnecessary when understanding the how and the why of connections between characters no longer matters.

Throughout the story, Lam examines the secondary pathologies of SARS, especially through mental illness and addiction. While in isolation with Chen, Fitz recounts a story of witnessing a resuscitation in a Kensington Market park, an episode that is likely the result of addiction (290–92). This moment of storytelling about an individual's health emergency balloons with symbolism in this story about mass contagion, as Lam questions exchanges between forms of suffering and relations between single and global emergencies. Fitzgerald has tremors and is suffering from alcohol withdrawal alongside SARS (275). He normally self-medicates for his nightmares with alcohol (277), and doesn't think to bring treatment for his withdrawal symptoms to the hospital where he is isolating (277), ironically demonstrating that the hospital is not a site that can always minister to all forms of suffering or medical need. His symptoms of alcohol withdrawal while in isolation are so severe that he suggests his supervising physician is writing up his case for a scientific publication entitled, "Tremor: A Novel Aspect of the SARS Syndrome" (287). As communities around the world discovered in 2020, the medical impacts of an epidemic go beyond the symptoms of the illness itself, and frequently increase rates of stress, mental illness, and addiction, as well as withdrawal symptoms.

Lam exposes how the physical impacts of addiction become wrapped up with the symptoms of epidemic disease. The supervising physician does finally prescribe withdrawal medication, but refuses to register Fitzgerald's Do Not Resuscitate request because he suspects it is spurred by mental illness, and he does not want to facilitate Fitzgerald's suicide (292–93). The lines blur between medicating for infectious disease and mental health, showing how the epidemic in fact causes overlapping illnesses. Lam explores another impact of SARS on the mental health of these characters in the nurse Dolores's panic attack as she flees before her shift, imagining she is ill (302–3). During both the SARS epidemic and COVID-19 pandemic, healthcare workers around the world suffered enormous assaults on their mental health, showing once more how epidemic illness can bring a broader array of pathologies beyond the symptoms of the initial disease.

As a form of diagnostic study, the story fetishizes the numbers that indicate the progression of the epidemic. "The next morning," Lam writes, "Fitz turned up his oxygen to fifteen litres per minute. He watched TV. SARS was now in Canada, Germany, Taiwan, China, Thailand, Hong Kong, Vietnam, and Singapore. The numbers seemed to grow by multiplication instead of addition" (280). The numbers measuring his oxygen, growing to match the rise in severity of his illness, parallel the increase in countries infected, and the observation of the mathematical rate of increase. In an epidemic, numbers become something to talk about. "Each day, the numbers on the television mounted," Lam writes. "One hundred and sixty-seven cases worldwide. Eight in Toronto. Thousands quarantined, and now the horrible, fascinating spectacle of new cases blooming, spreading, the numbers bursting bright on maps like dandelions on a mowed lawn after the rain" (272). This image of numbers as a spectacle of dandelions underscores the strange fascination digits take on in the face of contagion, while recalling that, as much as viruses spread death, they are also a form of life renewing itself. As Lam enumerates infected countries alongside oxygen counts and case numbers, the story focalizes how epidemics cause counting. The story closes with a news report observing that worldwide cases have "exceeded two thousand" with China alone announcing "three hundred and sixty-one new SARS cases and nine new deaths" (305). Epidemics make numbers something to talk about.

This interest in numbers recurs in other settings of Lam's story. Isolated, Fitzgerald counts time spent with others: "Seven minutes, was what he timed each day. Seven minutes of human contact in twenty-four hours" (271). The nurses are assigned to the SARS ward by a lottery (281), resulting in another numerical assignment of risk and luck that reduces meaning and life-or-death choices to number games. One reason for this intense focus on numbers is that mass contagion reduces all outcomes to a statistical threat, and people don't tend to be adept at calculating numerical risks. Lam dramatizes this challenge in a scene Chen and Fitzgerald remember witnessing, in which another physician persuades a patient to undergo an uncomfortable procedure to test for a one percent risk that she is suffering from a deadly condition. "One percent isn't bad" (295), she claims, reluctant, until the physician has her imagine that he is holding one of a hundred guns, one of which is loaded, saying, "The safety is off, shall I pull the trigger?" (296). Numerical risk is notoriously difficult for people to assess without such dramatizations to make it feel real, but the epidemic forces everyone to engage in such daily hypothetical number games. As the isolated doctors struggle to come to terms with their situation, they are left to wager on the risk of possible outcomes differentiated by their numerical scale: "If we die with only a few hundred others," says Fitzgerald.

> [W]e'll be SARS martyrs. If thousands get it but they find a cure and our deaths help, then it's worthwhile. If this thing just goes wild and the whole world dies by the millions, then we'll miss the worst of it. See? Can't lose.
>
> *(296)*

Assessing their risk from SARS means fitting themselves into possible scales of death tallies. In the end, Fitzgerald insists, outbreaks "run their course, they burn themselves out. It's just a question of how many people get burnt up in the process" (298). As the story makes clear throughout, this loaded numerical question of "how many" is the key source of drama and suspense in an epidemic.

Throughout the story, Lam foregrounds a variety of forms of reporting and documentation, which gives the tale a frame of historiographic metafiction, a feature Laura Moss also observes (21). As Linda Hutcheon famously establishes in *A Poetics of Postmodernism* (1988) and as I will discuss in greater depth in the next chapter, historiographic metafiction refers to work that self-consciously questions the relationship between fiction and history through an overt showcasing of the documents of both. In Lam's story, this tendency proceeds through an assembly of formal documents, from the supervising physician's dictated medical notes to file (272–74, 278–79, 292–93, 298–99), to the inclusion of the hospital's official "Addendum to SARS Bulletin 14" (299), to the reports on television (287) and the "Transcript of an evening news clip" from the CBC (304), and the World Health Organization (WHO) reports that open the story and that are then interspersed throughout (269–70, 272, 283, 287). In narrating this story through an archival gathering of potentially historical documents such as medical records and news reports, Lam is drawing attention to the contrasts between authoritative registers documenting the epidemic and the experience of the individuals suffering through it.

Comparing the doctor's notes to file with journalism about rising case counts, the news reports become case histories of a sick population. Lam's inclusion of doctors' files puts readers into the position of eavesdropping on medical care. In his notes, the consulting physician includes medical language, observing for example, "an O_2Sat of 88 percent," "Mild tachypnea," "air bronchograms suggestive of widespread consolidation," before listing the patient's medications: "We have continued the azithromycin, have added ceftriaxone, acyclovir, ribavirin, as well as a pulse course of solumedrol" (273). For most readers, this kind of medical language is meaningless, so they should question what Lam intends them to take from this cataloguing of terms. Part of the goal is to showcase how the language doctors use in response to crisis differs from the vocabularies of others, even as no language may fully explain calamity.

Lam's pile of documents and transcriptions raises the question of who is assembling all this info, for whom, and why, along with what the material is being positioned to prove. The authority that will make the final diagnosis of the meaning of all these events remains in question. The final elision of the nursing supervisor's retorts to Delores on their phone call (303–4) underscores this inaccessibility of authoritative viewpoints. Above all, the story offers its own record of contacts between the characters, its own contact tracing, and, in that sense, it positions both the reader and author as fulfilling an act of surveillance for the sake of public health. By putting itself up as a collection of historical documentation, this story questions the social impact of fiction itself.

Through this interest in documentation and reporting, Lam explores the role that the doctor plays in both ministering to and witnessing or documenting the ill, and the story examines this status through the role reversal of making the doctors themselves sick. Fitzgerald feels that "When he was alone in the room, he didn't want them to call him doctor, because it somehow implied that he should be partly floating above this illness and yet have some control over it" (270). The label of "doctor" is almost a costume, like a medical coat or mask, that denotes an alternate view of the scene. Lam's suggestion of the perspective of the doctor as "floating above this illness" but with "some control over it" positions the physician as a kind of omniscient narrator, or historian, someone with an almost disinterested perspective on the events. By infecting the doctors, Lam's story dismantles the idea that doctors can keep themselves apart from the calamities they witness: so long as the risk of contagion is there, either pathological or emotional, doctors risk becoming involved.

Speculative Contagion: Emily St. John Mandel's *Station Eleven* (2014)

One of the most popular new voices of Canadian literature in the twenty-first century, Emily St. John Mandel has twice trained her attention on speculative epidemics, in both *Station Eleven* (2014) and *Sea of Tranquility* (2022). Recalling Margaret Atwood's treatment of apocalyptic pandemic in *Oryx and Crake* (2003), *Station Eleven* portrays a "flu that exploded like a neutron bomb over the surface of the earth and the shock of the collapse that followed" (37). The novel tells the story of the outbreak by narrating its aftermath.

The book begins with the onstage cardiac death of an actor playing King Lear (7), an ironic end given the coming plague. As in Munro's work discussed previously, in times of mass mortality from disease, death from other causes becomes ironic. Beginning the story at the theatre, a scene of collective revelry soon to be made impossible by plague, also recalls Edgar Allan Poe's iconic story, "Masque of the Red Death" (1842), in which everyone dies when plague visits a ball. In work that follows such macabre dance of death traditions by framing mortality as a party, letting death rampage indiscriminately is a way to showcase the preciousness of life itself—a primary topic of Mandel's. The numbers quickly balloon to thirty-seven dead within two hours of the actor's death (22): the opening cardiac loss contrasts with the dozens of flu deaths that first night, a scale that itself hangs against the backdrop of the nearly terminal risk the disease poses to all of humanity.

The scenario of contrasting scales of death lets Mandel train her crystalline imagination on contemporary infrastructure, which her characters find an unlikely tenderness in remembering. "What was lost in the collapse," Mandel writes, "almost everything, almost everyone, but there is still such beauty" (57). Illness in this book is a device for exposing value in the mundane. To serve this goal, Mandel imagines a malady so lethal its death rate is nearly total. "The Georgia Flu was so efficient that there was almost no one left" (192), Mandel writes, and estimates of its mortality rate range from 99% to 99.99% (253, 61), ten times that of SARS and nearly a hundred times worse than COVID-19. The precise symptoms and progress of the illness are almost irrelevant given how quickly it kills. "Aches and pains. A sudden high fever. Difficulty breathing," an epidemiologist says, in response to a question about symptoms. "If you're exposed, you're sick in three or four hours and dead in a day or two" (235). The illness itself is hardly more than the rapid onset of death.

The extent of the threat is clear early on, but the characters struggle to grasp the full, world-destroying consequences of such a lethal pathogen.

In some ways the novel is a history of their effort to interpret the cataclysm. "It was possible to comprehend the scope of the outbreak," Mandel writes, "but it wasn't possible to comprehend what it meant" (236). From the beginning, trying to understand the illness involves contending with numerical data. A doctor reports case numbers from an emergency room on the first night of the outbreak: "A hundred and sixty in the past three hours. Fifteen of them have died. The ER's full of new cases. We've got beds parked in hallways. Health Canada's about to make an announcement" (18). The meaning of the epidemic is in its numbers, while the authority at hand, Health Canada, will always be behind the wave, always on the brink of making an announcement that will always be too late. Mandel imagines a pathogen advancing with exponential speed, leaving characters baffled: "How could so many die so quickly? The numbers seemed impossible" (176). Humanity has yet to encounter an illness with a total infection and mortality rate, but the terminal velocity of Mandel's imagined illness lets her put a frame around collective life and illustrate a hypothetical end point for the species.

Toronto's history with SARS offers a key backstory in this narrative of a new illness, as though Vincent Lam's characters in "Contact Tracing" survived to show up in Mandel's novel with their memories of the earlier outbreak intact. Jeevan's friend Hua calls him from the emergency room to warn him about the caseloads, because, he says, after the false scare of SARS, "You told me to call you if there was ever a real epidemic" (19). "It's the fastest incubation period I've ever seen," Hua says, urging Jeevan to leave the city. "You get exposed to this, you're sick within hours" (20). SARS also causes some sanguine initial responses to the virus that were echoed in Canadian communities during the emergence of COVID-19. "It'll be like SARS," says a cashier in response to Jeevan's load of disaster-prep groceries. "They made such a big deal about it, then it blew over so fast" (25), to which he replies, "This isn't like SARS. You should get out of the city" (25). The question of whether an illness is or is not like SARS has become a touchstone for Canadian attempts to interpret disease.

Whether or not they reference SARS, as Wendy Roy points out, many novels by Canadian women in the twenty-first century concern pandemics, from Atwood's *Oryx and Crake* (2003) and the rest of the *MaddAddam* series, but also works by less renowned writers, including Larissa Lai's *The Tiger Flu* (2018), and Saleema Nawaz's *Songs for the End of the World* (2020). Among these, Mandel's *Station Eleven* in particular, Roy suggests, displays the contagious circulation and impacts of texts, which can be as harmful as viruses, or present the salvation of a cure. Atasoy and Horan read how this communicative contagion in the novel spreads religiosity and connect it to Atwood's suggestion in *Oryx and Crake* that "Prayer had broken out" (qtd. in Atasoy and Horan 242). Mandel's thicket of references to Shakespeare's works have also drawn significant critical attention (see for example Herren; Lutz; Vermeulen).

Indeed, throughout the book, Shakespeare's life and work provide the characters with a parallel for their own calamity and a point of access to a culture that endures despite devastating illness. "Shakespeare had lived in a plague-ridden society with no electricity," Mandel writes, "and so did the Travelling Symphony" (288). Arthur dies while performing as King Lear (3–7), Kirsten plays Titania in *Midsummer Night's Dream* and reflects on its references to "rheumatic diseases" (58) and its composition "in 1594, the year London's theatres reopened after two seasons of plague" (57). The nomadic theatre company finds "that audiences seemed to prefer Shakespeare to their other theatrical offerings" because "People want what was best about the world" (38). Even as Shakespeare's artistry represents an enduring pinnacle of civilization, the characters are very aware of how his world resembled theirs. He lived a "plague-haunted life," and "was defined by" plague (308), but their experiences are also similar because of the lack of infrastructure. Mandel writes that "Plague closed the theatres again and again, death flickering over the landscape. And now in a twilight once more lit by candles, the age of electricity having come and gone, Titania turns to face her fairy king" (57). Shakespeare represents a creative force framed by illness and mortality, but also the cultural heights that are achievable within an elemental world without modern infrastructure.

Even though Mandel almost gleefully brings the species to the brink of extinction, what is most feared in this account is not the end of humanity, but the total loss of its facilities. The novel is resplendent with glistening descriptions of faltering infrastructure, as when Mandel writes that "The era of light pollution had come to an end. The increasing brilliance meant the grid was failing, darkness pooling over the earth" (251). The field of infrastructure studies has burgeoned in recent years (Pinnix et al.), and Tore Rye Andersen considers this focus through Mandel's interest in transparent commodities and the disrupted supply chain. The near-total destruction caused by the Georgia Flu gives Mandel the chance to regard infrastructure through a nostalgic lens, one that lavishes sentiment on objects that otherwise seem emotionless.

Mandel directs readers to the breadth of dismantlement in "An incomplete list" of the lost features of civilization that repeats a litany of "no more"—pools, flights, films, screens, and so on (31). This catalogue expressing the broken totality of world infrastructure ends with "No more avatars" (32). While this finale is an amusing reference to social media, the inclusion also recalls how this novel regards performance as preserving civilization itself, "Because," as in the travelling performers' motto, on its own, "survival is insufficient" (58). Questions of false, mistaken, and discovered identity, that is, avatars, recur through the book, as the Prophet's past as Arthur's son hovers beyond the avatar he's taken on as a dark mystic (280) and Clark realizes Kirsten performed in Arthur's final play (264). The illness both halts the roleplay of pre-pandemic civilization and permits new avatars afterwards. The opening death on stage, which Mandel circles for the rest of the novel, presages the coming onslaught of pandemic deaths, and can also be read as a signal that the play of contemporary civilization can no longer go on. Yet the play must go on and does in the theatrical resurrection of the travelling company, again, because survival is not sufficient. The claim "no more avatars," then, is both an astute gesture towards the masks of digital culture, and ironic, because the avatars of the stage in fact endure and condense as a key element of the survival of civilization in Mandel's vision.

The first category of infrastructure that Mandel's pandemic destroys is the healthcare system, as Health Canada's announcements can never catch up to the speed of the virus (17, 21) and hospitals are overwhelmed by the masses of arriving patients (18, 22). News stations persist heroically, as tearful broadcasters read reports (176), but Mandel chronicles their increasingly fragmented coverage (177) and eventual shuttering, as "countries began to go dark, city by city—no news out of Moscow, then no news out of Beijing, then Sydney, London, Paris, etc." (177). The silence of the news is echoed in the cessation of the audible drone of modern life: "Toronto was falling silent. Every morning the quiet was deeper, the perpetual hum of the city fading away" (177). Urban infrastructure can be heard vanishing.

Mandel gives Jeevan and Clark, the two adults who survive the onset of the pandemic, acute perspectives on the dismantling of infrastructure. Clark marvels at the lost "beauty of flight" (247), and the wonder of international telephone calls: "These taken-for-granted miracles that had persisted all around them" (233). Spurred by the memory of his lost curator boyfriend (254), Clark gathers objects to preserve and explain the marvels of the past in a museum (232), thereby reincarnating another form of public infrastructure. Clark focuses on the enduring physical remnants of vanished systems, such as iPhones and drivers' licences (254), both to build his museum and because "in his present state of mind, all objects were beautiful" (255). Jeevan in contrast fixates on cappuccinos as the sign of what he'll miss about civilization (174), considers "fires in a city without firefighters" (182), and "think[s] about how human the city is, how human everything is," in contrast to assumptions about "the impersonality of the modern world" (178). He realizes that "it had never been impersonal at all. There had always been a massive delicate infrastructure of people, all of them working unnoticed around us," without whom "the entire operation grinds to a halt" (178). This tender idea of "massive delicate infrastructure" is what is at stake in Mandel's apocalypse. The totally deadly illness gives Mandel a way to observe and write about the value of infrastructure. From cappuccinos to ID cards, the illness Mandel imagines opens a view of preciousness in the banal.

Shipping and cars become powerful emblems of the power of modern infrastructure. A character who works at a shipping company (80) marvels at the start of the pandemic that twelve percent of the world's ships are "moored fifty miles out of Singapore Harbour" (216) and she wonders if their workers are safe from the virus (227). Clark imagines the long sequence of now-vanished industry that produced a snow globe, from the designers and manufacturers to the shipping containers (255), and he muses about whether "somewhere there are ships setting out" (332). The interest in shipping containers proved prescient for the crisis of COVID-19, which caused major disruptions to the shipping industry, while shipping and its containers are a focus of the growing field of infrastructure studies in the humanities (see Klose). In this novel about global contagion, shipping gives Mandel another way to regard international circulation that parallels both the spread of disease and circuits within the body itself.

Mandel's macabre vision of the decay of infrastructure can also be seen in her frequent references to the cars that have become mausolea for pandemic victims. Because of how quickly the pandemic hits cities, highways are left full of cars after the collapse: "Traffic had inched along for the first two days, pulling trailers, plastic bins and suitcases strapped to roofs, but by the third morning the gridlock was absolute and people had started walking" (176). As a result, the wandering characters frequently come upon highways full of archaic cars. While hoping to rejoin her group, Kirsten discovers "miles of permanent gridlock" with "a skeleton in the driver's seat of the nearest car" (144); Jeevan passes "stopped cars with terrible things in them" (193); beyond the airport, the characters find only "abandoned cars as far as they could see, some with bodies inside" (256). The symbol of the car, reliant on the steel industry, shipping on a massive scale, and supply chains of gasoline and highway maintenance, is an emblem of human infrastructure that, in Mandel's vision, becomes a frame for human mortality.

Given the recurrence of cars and shipping in this story, it's significant that the best, most hopeful settlement, from which an electrified city can be seen on the horizon (311), is an airport—an ideal symbol of the sophisticated interconnectedness of the world before the plague. People start rebuilding society from this site of the pinnacle of society's accomplishments in technology and interconnection. The glimpse of a town with electric infrastructure returning (311) offers evidence of a long-term human triumph over the virus. Historic infrastructure becomes the subject of education in the postapocalyptic world, as children are taught about how "Satellites beamed information down to Earth. Goods travelled in ships and airplanes across the world" (262). Yet the new generation's "eyes glaze over when anyone talks to them about antibiotics or engines" (270), because these marvels of infrastructure exist only in a near-mythic past.

In an era of climate change, rather than offering the uneasy view of energy consumption that is now becoming common, this book honours machines, and doesn't address the environmental salvation a collapse might afford the earth itself. This reverence for contemporary infrastructure perhaps demarcates a shift in culture in the few years between this book's publication in 2014 and the COVID-19 pandemic, when many celebrated the resultant sudden drop in emissions. This context should direct how we interpret this story's fascination with infrastructure: in some ways *Station Eleven* is a profoundly conservative book because of the reverence it develops for what we might think of as the status quo. Mandel's elegiac gaze uses mourning to celebrate rather than critique modern humanity. For example, it is noteworthy that in a book concerned with land and nomadism in the Great Lakes area as colonial borders collapse, questions of Indigenous history, traditional knowledge, and precolonial trade routes and territory do not arise. Mandel ignores the colonial history that has given the landscape the place-names her characters work to remember, yet one wonders whether the routes the survivors find to navigate the region follow the footsteps of earlier people, an idea that I discuss in relation to Cherie Dimaline's *The Marrow Thieves* in my final chapter. In some senses, Mandel's novel represents a belated postcolonial explorer narrative that, through its reissuing of a colonial perspective, perpetuates the claim to the land of the dominant culture. By making these observations, I am not trying to suggest that Mandel should have written a different book, but I'm rather aiming to outline how the epidemic that she imagines permits the intensity of her celebratory focus on the world and its infrastructure *as it is*.

In Mandel's book, geography is reorganized and must be reconstructed due to the plague. The old circuits of landscape have been obliterated. Chicago is no longer a key mark on the map, but Kincardine, Ontario is. This rearrangement begins with the pandemic, and Mandel describes the few survivors always on the move early on, "before everyone caught on that there was no place they could walk to where life continued as it had before and settled wherever they could" (37). Two decades later Mandel writes, "they were still in motion, travelling back and forth along the shores of Lakes Huron and Michigan, west as far as Traverse City, east and north over the 49th parallel to Kincardine" (37). (This trajectory is hard to imagine, as Kincardine is in fact well south of the 49th parallel.)

As the illness reorganizes geography, places that were previously not likely to attract performers now do. The fictional town of St. Deborah by the Water marks "the southwestern border of the Symphony's territory, nothing much beyond it so far as anyone knew" (43). The desperate reports from Health Canada in the first days of the pandemic before its swift collapse (18, 21) expose the arbitrary character of national institutions much like borders. During Kirsten's walking escape from Toronto with her brother they travel "East and south. Around the lake and down into the United States. The border was open by then. All the guards had left" (188). The pandemic breaks down nation-states as much as bodies. The post-pandemic children struggle to conceive of this aspect of vanished infrastructure. "They were shown maps and globes, the lines of the borders that the Internet had transcended," Mandel writes. "That was Chicago. That was Detroit. The children understood dots on maps—*here*—but even the teenagers were confused by the lines. There had been countries, and borders. It was hard to explain" (262). Georgia flu is a disease that attacks geography itself.

In its study of illness, *Station Eleven* is not simply concerned with a mortal flu, but also portrays the state of postapocalyptic health and medicine. Not simply about the plague itself, the novel examines the global health implications of its aftermath, where a character fades away because she can no longer access antidepressants (242–45), where another dies because a nail in his foot gets infected (267), where bullets must simply be sewn up inside patients (272), where symptoms of post-traumatic stress disorder prevail (47) and characters are "plagued by nightmares" (304), where there is no anaesthetic (270). Early on, the characters consider the increase in risk from both illness and violence in the absence of modern medical interventions such as antibiotics and chemotherapy (253). Mandel focuses on Jeevan's process of sterilizing a needle with boiling water and moonshine (272). Once a paramedic, after training briefly with a former physician (271), he is now the "closest thing to a doctor in a one-hundred-mile radius" (270). Illnesses that are less fully deadly than the Georgia Flu also bedevil post-pandemic life: fevers hit St. Deborah by the Water (53, 126) and the Symphony (52), while Clark's closest friend dies "of an unknown illness in Year Seventeen" (276). The mortality rate of the Georgia Flu expands in the deaths from what would have previously been preventable causes.

Indeed, the illness gives narrative structure to the characters' lives. As the pandemic hits, Jeevan already feels that it will create "a *before* and an *after*, a line drawn through his life" (20). This idea of the illness causing narrative-like openings and closings recurs. Clark feels lucky not just to have evaded the virus, "but to have seen one world end and another begin"

(231). Kirsten summarizes the Prophet as "the bearer of another unfathomable story about walking out of one world and into another" (304). Stories trace connections between beginnings and endings, and the illness situates its victims and survivors within the same trajectory. The corrupted interpretation of this progression is that the impacts happen for a reason. As though in a metafictive reference to the narrative itself, the Prophet remarks that "all of your suffering, it's all part of a greater plan" (290), a phrasing repeated by the archer, who says that though "Some things in this life seem inexplicable . . . we must trust in the existence of a greater plan" (290). Illness can end and begin worlds, but the novel refuses the idea that its devastation has causal meaning, that it "happens for a reason" like a storyteller chooses plot points. Yet the wish to discern or impose causal narrative structure to the obvious before and after of the pandemic is a sympathetically human if toxic effort in this novel. Though narrative contains an explanatory impulse, part of what makes this book so compelling is the cool eye it casts on the inexplicability of both illness and civilization.

The question of causality is in fact one of the primary preoccupations of this novel, and one that links the mystery of contagious illness with the motives of narrative. As a precursor for the disorder of the pandemic, in the hours before his death Arthur experiences a "permanent state of disorientation like a low-grade fever, the question hanging over everything being How did I get from there to here?" (77). Answering the question raised by his illness would involve the rationalization of narrative. As the characters struggle to understand the meaning of the pandemic (236), its inexplicability breeds toxic interpretations. The villain of the book, the Prophet, leads a group that believe "they were saved from the Georgia Flu and survived the collapse because they're superior people and free from sin" (115), a belief that sanctifies the horrific violence they unleash against those who cross them (274). The Prophet has become dangerous because of his insistence on finding meaning in their apocalypse, and he repeats the idea that "everything that has ever happened on this earth has happened for a reason" (59, 253). Even as a child reading the Book of Revelation to a plane full of dead flu victims, he says, "I just want them to know that it happened for a reason" (259). His mother begins this trajectory by repeating her unexamined catchphrase that "Everything happens for a reason" (249, 261). The virulent disorder of his thinking is summarized as the problem that "He thinks the pandemic happened for a reason" (260). He describes the "perfection of the virus" over the "weak, inefficient viruses" that came earlier (60), viewing the Georgia Flu as an "avenging angel, unsurvivable" compared to the "trifling" illnesses against which they were vaccinated as children (60). He views the flu as a "cleansing" and, grasping to explain the inexplicable, suggests only the "pure" survived (60). The Prophet and his followers do not accept that the pandemic's dead were just "exposed to a certain virus, and we weren't" (259) as the only causal explanation that matters. While narrative tends to explain causes for events, *Station Eleven* gathers an ironic force in its insistence that nothing happens for a reason. Characters who believe otherwise are poisoned by the idea, in another kind of sickness or infection. As Dolores says, "That kind of insanity's contagious" (261).

When the COVID-19 pandemic hit during filming of the *Station Eleven* television series (Wetli), Mandel found herself on a press tour for *The Glass Hotel* (2020) (Waldman). All her appearances, suddenly by Zoom, were refocused on her now six-year-old novel, as its sales suddenly shot upward (Westenfeld). This scenario reflects the social life of a pandemic novel in a real time of illness. Mandel fictionalized the experience in *Sea of Tranquility* (2022), another novel about a pandemic. In that book, the idea of space travel gives Mandel a perspective from which the totality of earthly experience can be perceived, a view that the author achieves in the postapocalyptic rearview mirror of *Station Eleven*.

Conclusion

The works considered in this chapter show how epidemic illnesses never happen to one individual alone, but rather permeate social relations, and, as a result, change even geographies. As much as socializing spreads disease, plague impacts how people relate to each other. Spanning nearly two hundred years, these varied treatments of infectious diseases in Canadian literature show us how authors identify the broad social consequences of contagion.

Readers might find worthwhile points of comparison between Moodie's *Roughing It in the Bush* and *Station Eleven*. In both books, landscapes and towns are equally defined by the illnesses they contain or defend against. Both books overlook Indigenous claims to the land and could be productively read in relation to *The Marrow Thieves* by Cherie Dimaline (Métis), discussed in my fifth chapter. Whereas in Moodie's account, Canada itself comes into being as a landscape of potential contagion, a space of pathogenic risk, in Mandel's story, outbreak undoes the nation itself. While Moodie portrays a world devoid of the transit infrastructure Canadians have come to rely on, from trains to highways, Mandel imagines the aftermath of the collapse of these conveniences for people trying to navigate the same landscape. Moodie's world seems to resemble the one Mandel imagines as "an archipelago of small towns" that "fought off ferals, buried their neighbours, lived and died and suffered together" and "didn't go out of their way to welcome outsiders" (48). In both women's books, illness obstructs social relations, and Canada's landscape, so broad and so cold, magnifies those challenges, as the winter itself poses a physical threat to be survived. Both books show social relations occurring against a backdrop of contagion and pose the question of how people can collaborate to form productive communities in an environment where every conversation might breed death as much as survival—or delight.

Though illness indicates a calamity experienced by a particular body and can lead to medical isolation, in times of epidemic, we are never sick alone. This tenet will be underscored as we turn to the next chapter and consider Canadian literary depictions of the relation between disastrously injured characters and their caregivers.

Works Cited

Andersen, Tore Rye. "Snow Globes and Instant Coffee: Transparent Commodities and the Global Infrastructures of Late Capitalism in Contemporary Fiction." *Textual Practice*, vol. 38, no. 4, 2024, pp. 672–90.

Atasoy, Emrah, and Thomas Horan. "Prayer Had Broken Out: Pandemics, Capitalism, and Religious Extremism in Recent Apocalyptic Fiction." *Studies in the Novel*, vol. 54, no. 2, 2022, pp. 235–54.

Atwood, Margaret. *Oryx and Crake*. McClelland & Stewart, 2003.

Belshaw, John Douglas, et al. "Introduction: Framing an Accidental Past." *An Accidental History of Canada*, edited by Megan J. Davies and Geoffrey L. Hudson, McGill-Queen's, 2024.

The Bible. King James Version with the Apocrypha. 1611. Penguin, 2006.

Bolger, Francis W. P. *The Years before "Anne"*. Nimbus, 1991.

Braith, Melanie. "Braiding Stories, Braiding Kinship: How Cree Storytelling Restores Relationships in Tomson Highway's *Kiss of the Fur Queen*." *Canadian Literature*, no. 248, 2022.

Byrne, Katherine. *Tuberculosis and the Victorian Literary Imagination*. Cambridge UP, 2013.

Challacombe, L. "The Epidemiology of HIV in Canada." *CATIE—Canada's Source for HIV and Hepatitis C Information*, 24 Jan. 2024, www.catie.ca/the-epidemiology-of-hiv-in-canada.

Clark, Miriam Marty. "Allegories of Reading in Alice Munro's 'Carried Away'." *Contemporary Literature*, vol. 37, no. 1, 1996, p. 49.

Clement, Lesley D. "From 'Uncanny Beauty' to 'Uncanny Disease': Destabilizing Gender through the Deaths of Ruby Gillis and Walter Blythe and the Life of Anne Shirley." *L.M. Montgomery and Gender*, McGill-Queen's, 2021, pp. 44–67.

Closing Institutions for People with a Developmental Disability. Government of Ontario Newsroom, 31 Mar. 2009, www.news.ontario.ca/en/backgrounder/5213/closing-institutions-for-people-with-a-developmental-disability.

"Consumption, N., Sense 2.b." *Oxford English Dictionary*, Oxford UP, 2023.

Cook, Tim, and William Stewart. "War Losses (Canada)." *1914–1918 Online: International Encyclopedia of the First World War*, edited by Ute Daniel et al., Freie Universität Berlin, 2017.

CPSO. *Advice to the Profession: Maintaining Appropriate Boundaries*. College of Physicians and Surgeons of Ontario, www.cpso.on.ca/Physicians/Policies-Guidance/Policies/Boundary-Violations/Advice-to-the-Profession-Maintaining-Appropriate-B. Accessed 20 July 2024.

CPSO. *Boundary Violations Policy*. 2008. College of Physicians and Surgeons of Ontario, 2019, www.cpso.on.ca/Physicians/Policies-Guidance/Policies/Boundary-Violations.
CTV Ottawa. "Premier Wynne Apologizes to Former Residents of Rideau Regional Centre." *CTV News*, 17 Apr. 2014, www.ottawa.ctvnews.ca/premier-wynne-apologizes-to-former-residents-of-rideau-regional-centre-1.1780929.
Darroch, Heidi Tiedemann. "The War at Home: Writing Influenza in Alice Munro's 'Carried Away' and Kevin Kerr's Unity (1918)." *Canadian Literature*, no. 245, 2021, pp. 90–104, 192.
Daschuk, James W. *Clearing the Plains: Disease, Politics of Starvation, and the Loss of Aboriginal Life*. U of Regina P, 2013.
Decady, Yves, and Lawson Greenberg. *Ninety Years of Change in Life Expectancy*. Statistics Canada, July 2014, www150.statcan.gc.ca/n1/en/pub/82-624-x/2014001/article/14009-eng.pdf?st=0LqefWy8.
Duffin, Jacalyn. *History of Medicine: A Scandalously Short Introduction*. 3rd ed., U of Toronto P, 2021.
Duffin, Jacalyn. "Introduction: Lessons and Disappointments." *SARS in Context Memory, History, Policy*, edited by Jacalyn Duffin and Arthur Sweetman, McGill-Queen's, 2006, pp. 1–19.
Fahrni, Magda, and Esyllt W. Jones. "Introduction." *Epidemic Encounters: Influenza, Society, and Culture in Canada, 1918–20*, edited by Magda Fahrni and Esyllt W. Jones, U of British Columbia P, 2013, pp. 1–21.
Fiamengo, Janice. "'. . . The Refuge of My Sick Spirit . . .': L. M. Montgomery and the Shadows of Depression." *The Intimate Life of L. M. Montgomery*, edited by Irene Gammel, U of Toronto P, 2005, pp. 170–87.
Foucault, Michel. *The Birth of the Clinic: An Archaeology of Medical Perception*. 1963. Translated by A. M. Sheridan, Routledge, 1989.
Foxhall, Katherine. "Making Modern Migraine Medieval: Men of Science, Hildegard of Bingen and the Life of a Retrospective Diagnosis." *Medical History*, vol. 58, no. 3, 2014.
Fraile-Marcos, Ana María, and Lucía López-Serrano. "Stories as 'Med-Sins': Lee Maracle's *Ravensong* and *Celia's Song*." *Journal of Postcolonial Writing*, vol. 57, no. 6, Nov. 2021, pp. 738–51.
Gammel, Irene. "Reading to Heal: Anne of Green Gables as Bibliotherapy." *Anne's World: A New Century of Anne of Green Gables*, edited by Irene Gammel and Benjamin Lefebvre, U of Toronto P, 2010, pp. 82–99.
Ganz, Shoshannah. "Canadian Literary Representations of HIV/AIDS." *HIV in World Cultures*, edited by Gustavo Subero, Routledge, 2013, pp. 25–36.
Gillett, Margaret. "Abbott, Maude Elizabeth Seymour (Baptized Elizabeth Maud Seymour Babin)." *Dictionary of Canadian Biography*, vol. 16, U of Toronto P/Université Laval, 2016.
Glaze, Florence Eliza. "Medical Writer: 'Behold the Human Creature'." *Voice of the Living Light: Hildegard of Bingen and Her World*, edited by Barbara Newman, U of California P, 1998, pp. 125–49.
Grant, Kelly. "A Breath Atop the Mountain." *The Globe and Mail*, 30 Sept. 2023, p. A12.
Hallman, Stacey. "An Exploration of the Effects of Pandemic Influenza on Infant Mortality in Toronto, 1917–1921." *Canadian Studies in Population*, vol. 39, no. 3–4, 2013, p. 35.
Hammond, Mitchell. *Epidemics and the Modern World*. U of Toronto P, 2020.
Hands, Thora. *Drinking in Victorian and Edwardian Britain: Beyond the Spectre of the Drunkard*. Palgrave Macmillan, 2018.

Heidinger, Loanna. *Profile of Canadians Who Experienced Victimization during Childhood, 2018*. Statistics Canada, 12 Dec. 2022, www150.statcan.gc.ca/n1/pub/85-002-x/2022001/article/00016-eng.htm.
Herren, Graley. "The Prospero of Wonderland; Or, Miranda Carroll, Author of *Station Eleven*." *Comparative Drama*, vol. 57, no. 1–2, June 2023, pp. 139–64.
Highway, Tomson. *Kiss of the Fur Queen*. 1998. Penguin, 2021.
House, Tina. "Canada at the Bottom of G7 Nations in Fight against HIV." *Aboriginal Peoples Television Network*, 24 Apr. 2024, www.aptnnews.ca/national-news/canada-at-the-bottom-of-g7-nations-in-fight-against-hiv.
Humphries, Mark Osborne. *The Last Plague: Spanish Influenza and the Politics of Public Health in Canada*. U of Toronto P, 2012.
Hutcheon, Linda. *A Poetics of Postmodernism: History, Theory, Fiction*. Routledge, 1988.
Jamieson, Sara. "*Âyahkwê* Songs: AIDS and Mourning in Gregory Scofield's 'Urban Rez' Poems." *Canadian Poetry*, vol. 57, Fall 2005, pp. 52–64.
Johnston, Julie. *Hero of Lesser Causes*. Lester, 1992.
Kang, Nancy. "Pray, Then Prey: Reconstituting the Cree Weetigo Story in Tomson Highway's *Kiss of the Fur Queen*." *LIT Literature Interpretation Theory*, vol. 28, no. 3, July 2017, pp. 195–216.
Klose, Alexander. *The Container Principle: How a Box Changes the Way We Think*. Translated by Charles Marcrum II, MIT, 2015.
Krotz, Sarah Wylie. "Productive Dissonance: Classical Music in Tomson Highway's *Kiss of the Fur Queen*." *Studies in Canadian Literature*, vol. 34, no. 1, Jan. 2009, pp. 182–203.
Lam, Vincent. "Contact Tracing." *Bloodletting & Miraculous Cures*, Anchor, 2005, pp. 269–306.
Lecker, Robert. "Machines, Readers, Gardens: Alice Munro's 'Carried Away." *Essays on Canadian Writing*, vol. 66, 1998, pp. 103–27.
Ledwell, Jane, and Jean Mitchell. "Introduction." *Anne Around the World: L. M. Montgomery and Her Classic*, edited by Jane Ledwell and Jean Mitchell, McGill-Queen's, 2013, pp. 3–27.
Lefebvre, Benjamin, editor. *The L. M. Montgomery Reader: Volume One: A Life in Print*. U of Toronto P, 2020.
Leggatt, Judith. "Raven's Plague: Pollution and Disease in Lee Maracle's *Ravensong*." *Mosaic*, vol. 54, no. 2, 2021, pp. 73–87.
Library and Archives Canada. *Archived—Julie Johnston*, 29 May 2001, www.collectionscanada.gc.ca/read-up-on-it/015020-6043-e.html.
Lutz, Michael. "'The Promised End': Shakespeare and Extinction." *Variable Objects: Shakespeare and Speculative Appropriation*, edited by Valerie M. Fazel and Louise Geddes, Edinburgh UP, 2021, pp. 230–47.
Mandel, Emily St. John. *Sea of Tranquility*. Picador, 2023.
Mandel, Emily St. John. *Station Eleven*. HarperCollins, 2014.
Maracle, Lee. *Ravensong*. Press Gang, 1993.
Mawdsley, Stephen E. "Borders and Blood Fractions: Gamma Globulin and Canada's Fight against Polio, 1950–55." *Canadian Bulletin of Medical History*, vol. 36, no. 2, 2019, pp. 444–68.
McCuaig, Katherine. *Weariness, the Fever, and the Fret: The Campaign Against Tuberculosis in Canada, 1900–1950*. McGill-Queen's, 1999.
Miles, Steven H. *The Hippocratic Oath and the Ethics of Medicine*. Oxford UP, 2005.
Montgomery, Lucy Maud. *Anne of Green Gables*. 1908. Aladdin, 2001.
Montgomery, Lucy Maud. *Anne of the Island*. 1915. Seal, 1996.
Montgomery, Lucy Maud. *Emily of New Moon*. 1925. Seal, 1983.

Moodie, Susanna. *Roughing It in the Bush*. 1852. McLelland & Stewart, 1989.
"Mortality Analyses." *Johns Hopkins Coronavirus Resource Center*, 16 Mar. 2023, www.coronavirus.jhu.edu/data/mortality.
Moss, Laura. "'A Science of Uncertainty': Bioethics, Narrative Competence, and Turning to the 'What if' of Fiction." *Studies in Canadian Literature*, vol. 40, no. 2, 2015, pp. 5–24.
Munro, Alice. "Carried Away." *Open Secrets*, Penguin, 1994, pp. 1–59.
Negin, Joel, et al. "HIV among Indigenous Peoples: A Review of the Literature on HIV-Related Behaviour since the Beginning of the Epidemic." *AIDS and Behavior*, vol. 19, no. 9, 2015, pp. 1720–34.
Neilson, Shane. "Public Health Disruptions in Susanna Moodie's *Roughing It in the Bush* and Catharine Parr Traill's *The Backwoods of Canada*." *Studies in Canadian Literature*, vol. 48, no. 1, 2023, pp. 87–108.
Olaveson, Heather. "'Coming Home' Through Music: Cree and Classical Music in Tomson Highway's *Kiss of the Fur Queen*." *Canadian Literature*, no. 232, Spring 2017, pp. 65–80.
Pike, E. Holly, and Laura M. Robinson. "'You Don't Want Me Because I'm Not a Boy': L. M. Montgomery and Gender." *L. M. Montgomery and Gender*, edited by E. Holly Pike and Laura M. Robinson, McGill-Queen's, 2021, pp. 1–17.
Pinnix, Aaron, et al., editors. *Rethinking Infrastructure Across the Humanities*. transcript Verlag, 2023.
Piper, Liza. *When Disease Came to This Country: Epidemics and Colonialism in Northern North America*. Cambridge UP, 2023.
Poe, Edgar Allan. "The Masque of the Red Death." *The Portable Edgar Allan Poe*. 1842, Penguin, 2006, pp. 37–43.
Pormohammad, Ali, et al. "Comparison of Confirmed COVID-19 with SARS and MERS Cases—Clinical Characteristics, Laboratory Findings, Radiographic Signs and Outcomes: A Systematic Review and Meta-Analysis." *Reviews in Medical Virology*, vol. 30, no. 4, July 2020, p. e2112.
Prycer, Melissa. "The Hectic Flush: The Fiction and Reality of Consumption in L. M. Montgomery's Life." *The Intimate Life of L. M. Montgomery*, edited by Irene Gammel, U of Toronto P, 2005, pp. 258–73.
Robertson, David A. *Scars*. HighWater, 2010.
Roy, Wendy. "Trauma and the Ethics of Literary Culture in the Time of Pandemic: Emily St. John Mandel's *Station Eleven* and Saleema Nawaz's *Songs for the End of the World*." *Studies in Canadian Literature*, vol. 47, no. 1, Dec. 2022, pp. 50–72.
Rubio, Mary Henley. *Lucy Maud Montgomery: The Gift of Wings*. Doubleday, 2008.
Scofield, Gregory. *Native Canadiana: Songs from the Urban Rez*. Polestar, 1996.
"Settlement Reached in Rideau Regional Class-Action Lawsuit." *CBC News*, 24 Dec. 2013, www.cbc.ca/news/canada/ottawa/settlement-reached-in-rideau-regional-class-action-lawsuit-1.2475215.
Simpson, Leanne Betasamosake. *As We Have Always Done: Indigenous Freedom through Radical Resistance*. U of Minnesota P, 2017.
Skinner, Andrea Robin. "My Stepfather Sexually Abused Me When I Was a Child: My Mother, Alice Munro, Chose to Stay with Him." *Toronto Star*, 7 July 2024.
Sopiarz, Josh. "Hostess, Ghost, and Apocalypse: Reconsidering Alice Munro's 'Carried Away'." *The American Review of Canadian Studies*, vol. 51, no. 2, 2021, pp. 237–50.
Statistics Canada. *Life Expectancy, 1920–1922 to 2009–2011*, 15 Feb. 2016, www150.statcan.gc.ca/n1/pub/11-630-x/11-630-x2016002-eng.htm.

Stiles, Anne. *Children's Literature and the Rise of "Mind Cure": Positive Thinking and Pseudo-Science at the Fin de Siècle*. Cambridge UP, 2020.
Vermeulen, Pieter. "Beauty That Must Die: *Station Eleven*, Climate Change Fiction, and the Life of Form." *Studies in the Novel*, vol. 50, no. 1, 2018, pp. 9–25.
Waldman, Katy. "The Rewriting of Emily St. John Mandel." *The New Yorker*, Apr. 2022, www.newyorker.com/culture/persons-of-interest/the-rewriting-of-emily-st-john-mandel.
Westenfeld, Adrienne. "Emily St. John Mandel Is Nobody's Prophet." *Esquire*, 13 Dec. 2021.
Wetli, Patty. "In Eerie Coincidence, HBO's Flu Pandemic, Post-Apocalyptic Series 'Station Eleven' Filming in Chicago." *WTTW*, 6 Feb. 2020.
WHO. *Summary of Probable SARS Cases with Onset of Illness from 1 November 2002 to 31 July 2003*. World Health Organization, 24 July 2015, www.who.int/publications/m/item/summary-of-probable-sars-cases-with-onset-of-illness-from-1-november-2002-to-31-july-2003.
WHO Health Emergencies Programme. *COVID-19 Deaths: WHO COVID-19 Dashboard*. World Health Organization, www.data.who.int/dashboards/covid19/cases. Accessed 22 July 2024.
Williamson, Bess. *Accessible America: A History of Disability and Design*. New York UP, 2019.

2

DISASTROUS INJURY AND THE RECUPERATION OF HISTORY IN POSTMODERN NOVELS

This chapter examines how massive injury in postmodern Canadian literature represents the obstructions to language and history posed by war and trauma. Resurrecting narrative from ruined bodies often falls to caregivers in these books, so that working at the bedsides of injured people becomes a means of preserving history. In such works about trauma, the destruction of the body parallels the social impacts of war and illuminates the stakes of storytelling and history itself. The doctor or caregiving storyteller became a familiar trope through the social media reporting of practitioners in the COVID-19 pandemic (see Al-Rawi and Zemenchik; Ford et al.), but this tradition in Canadian literature has long roots, and examining this figure will contribute to this chapter's discussion of how the destroyed body often represents a ruptured sense of history.

The chapter begins with Timothy Findley's *The Wars* (1977), moving to Joy Kogawa's *Obasan* (1981) followed by the signal text for exploring this theme in Canadian literature, Michael Ondaatje's *The English Patient* (1992), before closing with Shani Mootoo's *Cereus Blooms at Night* (1996). These stories about severely injured people exhibit a recursive preoccupation with the impacts of war and violence and reveal the postmodern feeling that once-unspeakable ruptures can be talked about, an opening of expression and representation often made possible by a fragmentary style. Alongside their reconstructions of history and their portrayals of relationships between patients and caregivers, these books present pain as an experience that troubles narrative representation, that prompts and defies telling.

I have chosen to highlight the books discussed in this chapter for how they illustrate postmodernism, the challenges to literary representation

DOI: 10.4324/9781003340119-3

posed by the calamities of the twentieth century, and the genre of the historical novel. Treated at greater length than the other novels, this chapter also seeks to contextualize the major significance of *The English Patient* as perhaps the preeminent Canadian illness narrative. The books I have chosen to accompany it here advance that goal. These are not the only Canadian novels about wounds, however, and both earlier and later works concern disastrous injury. Hugh MacLennan's historical account of the 1917 Halifax Explosion in *Barometer Rising* (1941) offers an early examination of a catastrophe that caused widespread death and destruction on Canadian soil. David Bergen's *The Time in Between* (2005) examines a character suffering from post-traumatic stress decades after participating in the Vietnam War. *Invisible Injured* (2017), a Canadian history of traumatic injury in conflict zones by medical historian Adam Montgomery, and *After the War* (2018), his book on post-traumatic stress syndrome co-authored with Stéphane Grenier, also offer context for Canadian narrative about the meaning of disastrous injury, its care, and its stories.

Although these novels concern the narration of the past, they should not be read as factual depictions of historical injury but rather as works of representation that use the idea of massive wounds to explore the conditions of communication despite trauma. While *Obasan* relates the near-destruction of the protagonist's mother in the 1945 atomic bombing of Nagasaki, and *Cereus Blooms at Night* narrates the lasting injury of sexual violence, both *The English Patient* and *The Wars* present characters suffering from full-body burns. Without antibiotics and other modern advancements in burn care that emerged during and after World War II, most victims of such overwhelming injuries would quickly succumb to infection (Lee et al.). As a result, the idea of a figure alive but suffering from near-total burns in both these novels should be read as a somewhat anachronistic fantasy that serves metaphorical rather than documentary goals. Rather than being simple windows to past suffering, these works problematize historical narration itself.

Postmodernism, Historiographic Metafiction, and the Historical Novel

The cluster of books I discuss in this chapter reflect the late-twentieth-century postmodern turn in art and literature, which is characterized by an increased interest in fragmented forms of representation and subjective historical interpretation (see Hutcheon, *Poetics* 89–90). These books evince postmodernism not only in the two-decade period of their publication, but also in their style, their thematic concerns, and in how they reward readings through postmodern critical theory. Ondaatje, Kogawa, and

Mootoo's works reflect postcolonial readings of literature (see for example Marais; McGonegal 111–47, and Saeed, respectively), while Mootoo's and Findley's invite interpretation through queer theory (see O'Callaghan; Facundo 129–49). In short, though these books stand as major works in the Canadian canon for this time period and reflect the themes of affliction, storytelling, and caregiving that I am exploring here, they also serve as representative texts for understanding important interpretive frameworks in literary criticism that emerged in the late twentieth century.

In questioning what it means to speak of pain and the significance of silence, these books echo the concerns of many postmodern literary theorists. Elaine Scarry considers these questions in relation to torture and notions of reality in *The Body in Pain* (1985), while Susan Sontag examines the stakes of looking at such depictions in *Regarding the Pain of Others* (2003). Another key interpretive angle for this fiction is the notion of trauma, whose invitations and barriers to narration and history Cathy Caruth explores through the lens of psychoanalysis. Since the English patient's destroyed body is a symbol of the fate of history during and after World War II, his physical tragedy parallels Kogawa's description of Naomi's mother's injury in the atomic bombing of Nagasaki. Both destroyed bodies represent the civilization-ending cataclysm of World War II. In both books, the dropping of atomic bombs signals a horizon for human pain and destruction, an outer limit beyond which horror becomes incomprehensible, unavailable to human knowledge and therefore to narration. As Michael Rothberg explains, many theorists of postmodern culture explore this concept of unspeakable atrocity in relation to World War II and the Holocaust, including Jean-François Lyotard, Maurice Blanchot, and Theodor Adorno, who continuously returned to and reconsidered his famous 1951 suggestion that "To write poetry after Auschwitz is barbaric" (see Rothberg 25–58). Spurred partly by the calamity of the AIDS epidemic, by the late-1990s moment of Shani Mootoo's publication of *Cereus Blooms at Night*, the techniques and ways of looking at the world that had helped earlier postmodern authors narrate the horrors of the World Wars were increasingly available for use in expressing other previously unspeakable feelings, such as gender questioning and queer desire (see Kruger). These novels can thus be put into conversation with postmodern literary theory through their concern with the limits of narrating both physical and emotional pain and questions regarding how silence harms or cures.

Theories of the historical novel also offer a key critical context for these works. Historical novels let authors narrate prior social moments that often have established narratives in popular consciousness. Writing in the 1930s, the influential Marxist literary theorist Georg Lukács explained the development of the historical novel with reference to works by nineteenth-century authors including Sir Walter Scott and Leo Tolstoy. Lukács suggests that the genre often focalizes national conflict through the experiences of an individual protagonist, thereby illustrating national historical struggles at both intimate and grand social scales. Findley and Ondaatje's works fit within this framework, as they each follow the lives of individual Canadians through their wartime experiences. Kogawa's semi-autobiographical text can also be read through this lens but represents a more complex use of the genre since rather than shoring up the authority of the Canadian state, it uses the individual perspective of the narrator to question the attack of that state on one of its own communities. The postmodern turn impacts the genre of the historical novel by making the status of knowledge about the past part of the topic of fiction, as these works demonstrate through their overt focus on archival documents.

This concern reflects a final relevant branch of critical theory regarding postmodern representations of history—Linda Hutcheon's famous notion of historiographic metafiction. Works that exhibit this feature of much postmodern narrative in Canada self-consciously foreground the fragmented assembly of history from often-scattered documents, so that, as Hutcheon explains, "The epistemological question of how we know the past joins the ontological one of the status of the traces of that past" (*Poetics* 122). In a foundational discussion of the concept in *The Canadian Postmodern* (1988), Hutcheon notes that *The Wars* and *Obasan* both reflect this tendency. Published later, *The English Patient* and *Cereus Blooms at Night* also exhibit the assimilation of historical documents into the genre of the novel as a way of recuperating the past.

This recuperative process can be connected to Arthur W. Frank's ideas about how the experience of suffering prompts and conditions narrative. As Frank notes, the mythic figure of the wounded healer is also often a wounded storyteller (xii). All these books could be read within Frank's category of stories prompted by wounds, as ruptures of the body and its care call for narration, even as they also often demonstrate the insufficiencies of language, and the challenge of reconstituting the past from its physical remnants.

The works under discussion here exemplify how postmodern authors have confronted failures of language in response to the atrocities of war, racism, gender-based discrimination, and sexual violence, and found ways to tell of the broad social impacts of these histories through the suffering of individuals and their caregivers. As we shall see, the effort to recuperate history in these books travels through the effort to rehabilitate severely injured people.

Timothy Findley's *The Wars* (1977)

Published fifteen years before *The English Patient* but now less-often remembered, Timothy Findley's *The Wars* (1977) won the Governor General's Award and bears striking similarities to the newer, more famous novel, both in its treatment of world war, and its notion of fragmented history. Like *The English Patient*, the book presents itself as a collection of documents and testimonies from various witnesses to the main events. Findley's poetic and fragmentary style is often strongly evocative of Ondaatje's approach, and some lines of Findley's would not be out of place in the later book, for example when he writes, "As the past moves under your fingertips, part of it crumbles" (9), or describes how a burning man "leaps through memory without a sound. The archivist sighs. Her eyes are lowered above some book. . . . You lay the fiery image back in your mind and let it rest" (11). The parallels between the themes and styles of these two novels offer students and their instructors scope for fruitful comparisons, as well as considerations of literary influence.

The Wars recounts layers of catastrophic injuries among human and animal participants in and bystanders of World War I. Nonchronological and multivocal, the novel represents an effort to set the individual story of the soldier Robert Ross against the broad historical narrative of World War I. Engaging with the many scholarly discussions of Findley's portrayal of photographs as documentary evidence including Lorraine York's, David Williams suggests that *The Wars* should be read for its framing of history and historicism, and, as mentioned previously, the book offers a classic example of what Linda Hutcheon calls historiographic metafiction. Near total injury here as in *The English Patient* and *Obasan* represents both the desire for and the inaccessibility of knowledge about the past.

Illness, injury, and their care make up substantial portions of Findley's book, but above all the author frames the physical pain of World War I through its attacks on animal welfare, the stakes of which Peter Webb considers in detail. A main plot point of the novel, Robert's concern for the welfare of war horses, originates because of the sickness of their usual caregiver (56): "It was because of Harris's illness that Robert became involved with the horses" (57). This involvement with animals is the unexpected primary theme of this war novel. Robert goes to war because he doesn't want to kill the pet rabbits of his dead sister (20–26). At the end of his time in service, he breaks ranks to defy Captain Leather's order not to free forty horses and mules on the brink of being shelled to death (185–86), euthanizes the dying animals, and shoots Leather himself, before "he tore the lapels from his uniform and left the battlefield" (186). Robert's time as a soldier, a hired gun, is bookended by his refusals to permit animals' needless suffering, offering a stark parallel to the vast human pain inflicted by war itself.

Findley's novel offers numerous scenes of historical interest regarding hospitals and medical care, such as a rendition of a ward of the Royal Free Hospital in London (94), and a description of how a large country house turns into an infirmary. In Lady Juliet's account, St Aubyn's, Lady Emmeline's country home, "became much more than a haven for her sons and an anchor for her daughter," because, as the war gets worse, "a flood of Clive and Barbara's friends in need of rest began to give the place the feel of a hostel" (148). Recognizing the need at hand, Lady Emmeline has her husband arrange for "a charter declaring St Aubyn's a convalescent hospital" (148). In this vignette, the hospital represents an outgrowth of the social world of the British upper classes, as medical benevolence replaces the social triumph of popularity, and friends' visits turn into patient stays. The medical horror of war is encapsulated in a scene at the front, where, amid the carnage, "One man lay alive on a stretcher while at either end the stretcher bearers curled like caterpillars—dead" (120). This image, one of the most poignant in the book, encapsulates the stark and tragic perspective on wartime medical care that Findley develops throughout the book.

As befitting a novel about World War I, the book rebounds with deaths, not simply in trenches, but in hospitals and at home. As the narrator writes towards the end of the novel, "So far, you have read of the deaths of 557,017 people—one of whom was killed by a streetcar, one of whom died of bronchitis and one of whom died in a barn with her rabbits" (164). Characters are systematically mutilated until they die, in torments that reflect what the war does to animals and that show its meaningless destruction. Many men languish in hospital, and foreshadow Robert's own ending, totally burned and wrapped in medical dressings. While visiting a friend in hospital, Robert witnesses two acquaintances, Taffler and Barbara, visiting "a man entirely encased in bandages. He was quite unable to move. Robert had already been intrigued by his silence" (97). Taffler leans down and whispers something that "went unheard by anyone except the man in the bandages" to which "he was straining to reply—but no words came: not even a whisper" (97). Robert "could feel the man in the bandages 'screaming' and the sensation of this silent agony at the other end of the room was finally so strong that Robert had to go and get one of the nurses," who gives him some morphine (98). The bandaged man, Villiers, it emerges, "had been trapped in a fire and his vocal cords destroyed when he'd swallowed the flames" (98). This scene of a man so burned that speaking or not speaking depends on morphine anticipates *The English Patient*, and shows how Canadian authors have imagined how the extremities of war impact language and the possibility of verbal communication. If the atrocity of war is unspeakable, writers can dramatize that challenge to expression in characters so damaged they cannot speak.

Findley's novel returns again and again to scenes of men left alive only for despair and driven to extremity by romantic frustration and their apocalyptic injuries. The agony Taffler inflicts on Villiers is turned on himself when he loses both arms, and receives a visit from Robert and Barbara, now romantically involved themselves and so repeating the stress Taffler inflicted on Villiers before. Taffler has lost both arms and, in one of the novel's most perverse scenes, Lady Juliet comes upon him trying to die by stripping bandages with his teeth (157) and "rubbing his wounds to make them bleed. The stumps where his arms had been were raw and one of them was pumping blood in spurts across the floor" (158). That both scenes of agony are prompted by the men's frustration over visits from the same woman with whom they are both in love shows Findley amalgamating romantic and physical desperation and pain.

These vignettes foreshadow the suffering of Robert himself, who, burned nearly to death, becomes the novel's third totally bandaged man. He is seen in this condition primarily through interviews with Marian Turner, "a nurse in the Great World War" who "remembers Robert vividly. It was she who received him and cared for him after he'd been arrested and brought into the hospital" (13). The novel opens and closes with transcripts of her interviews. She says she assumed Robert was "extremely well made" though "because of what happened I can't remark about the face" (14). She is very struck by "the way he was—the burns—the pain and the dreadful, dreadful silence that surrounded him" (196). As in *The English Patient*, this scene of care for a patient beyond their initial total burning is not realistic, as without antibiotics patients with such injuries quickly die of infection. The scene rather serves Findley's literary motives. The nurse is taken with Robert, and says, "I could speak to him—and I often did—but I didn't expect replies, except this once" (196), because, she says, "I wanted to help him die" (196). This desire, prompted by admiration for her patient, runs counter to her professional training: "I'm a nurse. I've never offered death for anyone" but in this moment she "wanted to offer some way out of life—I wanted grace for Robert Ross" (196–97). His two-word response closes out their exchange and his life story: "Not yet" (197). This scene will gain relevance in the discussion of medical assistance in dying (MAID) in the next chapter, and readers might connect it to Miriam Toews's *All My Puny Sorrows*. As in *The English Patient* too, caregiving offers a privileged position from which to learn—and potentially end—a patient's story. That the novel concludes with Marian's perspective on Robert's own final days (194–95) makes her portrait of him seem almost decisive, the final word. The patient's story becomes the caregiver's story.

Findley frames *The Wars* as an archivist's attempt to gather Robert's history, but in this effort, nurses and archivists hold similar positions, and it's important to regard the overt historiographic metafiction of this book in relation to its interest in medical care. Findley opens his novel with the idea of being at an archive, with documents and pictures "Spread over table tops, a whole age lies in fragments underneath the lamps" (9). The novel's status as a splicing together of paper artefacts makes the actual word-for-word repetition of the prologue towards the end of the book (190) readable as yet another document slid between Findley's pages. At the end, he writes, declaring Robert's story over, "The archivist closes her book" (200). Findley aligns the shadowy figure of the archivist, history's steward, with the nurse, the patient storyteller's guardian.

This novel is overtly concerned with the memories of nurses, attendants to the dying. "All of this happened a long time ago," Findley writes.

> But not so long ago that everyone who played a part in it is dead. Some can still be met in dark old rooms with nurses in attendance. They look at you and rearrange their thoughts. They say: "I don't remember." The occupants of memory have to be protected from strangers.
>
> *(8)*

There is a slippage here between those who remember and the nurses who attend them, and Findley is likely purposefully ambiguous about whether he intends the distinction or not. Nurses are party to more secrets of their patients than they have a right to disclose to others. Once more we see the professionalized idea of taking a medical history, the storytelling that transpires between caregiver and patient, aligned with the meaning of storytelling from the brink of death.

This comparison of archivists and nurses aligns hospitals and libraries as public institutions. Yet these civic spaces are differentiated by the relative privacy of the stories they hold. "Then the nurses nod at you," Findley writes, "much as to say—you see? It's best to go away and find your information somewhere else. In the end, the only facts you have are public" (8). The scene of care in hospitals both is public, and isn't, representing the individual patient's private pain and, often, encounter with death. Above all, recuperating history in this book is tied to the effort to help others recuperate.

Joy Kogawa's *Obasan* (1981)

Joy Kogawa's *Obasan* (1981) also chronicles the near obliteration of a person, and the questions about aftermath that result. This influential work explores the perspective of Naomi in adulthood as she looks back on her childhood suffering during the 1940s internment of Japanese Canadians. She longs for her mother who vanished in Japan, experiences sexual abuse by a neighbour, and witnesses the traumatized silence of her grandmother, Obasan, and the dogged search for answers of her aunt, Emily. Naomi eventually learns that her mother was horrifically injured in the bombing of Nagasaki, a destruction of an individual that parallels the racist attack on a whole community during the internment that the book also documents. As Diana Brydon suggests, the book "describes the Canadian nation at a time of great collective sickness," with "the disease of racism infecting the body politic," and both literally sickening and forcing Naomi's family, through "[t]heir insistence on mattering," to be "part of the cure" (466). In presenting historical insights into the racism of the internment and cultures surrounding doctors and hospitals, Kogawa's novel shows that silence itself is also an injury and that storytelling can soothe pain.

In this novel, doctors are privileged figures who cause both hope and bad news, while hospitals represent a social space that coalesces many forces of racism and isolation. The story begins with a doctor's call, bringing news of Naomi's uncle's death (13). Death, and a doctor's message, give this narrative its starting place. Naomi's grandfather is a doctor, whose status allows him to visit the prison known as "the Pool" (89), the Hastings Park internment camp where eight thousand Japanese Canadians were detained in 1942 (Robinson 135). He falls ill after visiting a sick patient (85), but Emily writes that his concern for the welfare of his community, as well as the limp and cough of his son-in-law and grandson, make him "a terrible patient" (87). "A lot of his patients, especially the old ones," she writes, "are in a state of collapse" (87). The extreme physical burden of the internment cannot be overstated, and represents the broader health impacts of racism, which by now are well documented (see Nestel). A variety of hospitals feature in this work and stand as parallel institutions to the racist internment centre in Vancouver. Naomi's father and paternal grandfather are separated from the family in hospital (129), and she herself is hospitalized after nearly drowning (136). While recuperating she has a nightmare that ties many bad experiences to the space of the hospital (136). Her father dies in hospital after his last letter mentions his treatment by a "doctor he doesn't trust" (183), confirming Naomi's earlier observation that "Hospitals are places where Death visits" (138). Far from being a simple symbol of medical care, the institution of the hospital parallels the spectre of the internment camp and represents the scene of one of Naomi's greatest losses.

The social impacts of this experience are presented as physical wounds. Emily positions the legacy of the nation's internment of Japanese Canadians as a self-inflicted injury, saying, "What this country did, it did to itself" (34). The book uncovers economic motivations for the political attacks on the community, which gave white Canadians an excuse to take the livelihoods and assets of those they expelled from their homes (77). A news article about how the exiled Canadians may not return to the British Columbia coast for another year though the war is long over blames the racism of locals: their leaders thought "the government was wise in giving the old sores another year to heal" (181). This is a terrible justification for continuing the harm of their expulsion long after the purported political reasons for the policy have ended. Naomi points out the absurdity of this claim, writing, "Another year? Which year should we choose for our healing?" (181). Even after the restrictions are lifted, she writes, "the 'old sores' remain. In time the wounds will close"—but they haven't yet (181). The experience of the racist interment policy is itself an injury that does not heal.

In a moment that devastates Naomi, the children at the public bath say they are shunning her and her family because "You're sick. You've all got TB. . . . That's why Stephen is limping" (151). Much as the harm of the internment is a kind of wound, illness is presented as an excuse for prejudicial social striation within the exiled community. The experience prompts Naomi's uncle to explain to her that "For some people it is a shameful matter to be ill. But it is a matter of misfortune, not shame" (151). Kogawa layers illnesses and wounds upon each other, providing explanations for and causes of misfortune and shame and diagnosing sources of injury within the nation, the Japanese-Canadian community, Naomi's family, and her experiences.

The search for explanations also carries medical and physical connotations. While Naomi is "Devoured alive" and "consumed by the question" of what her mother was like, "The past hungers" for Obasan, "feasts on her" (28). These consumption metaphors for the characters' relationships to the past make their longing physical. Early on the narrator describes her Aunt Emily, who hunts for information about what her family and community went through during the internment, as "one of the world's white blood cells, rushing from trouble spot to trouble spot with her medication pouring into wounds" (35). Knowing and uncovering the truth here stands in for the biological function of the immune system, providing a cure. Recalling *The English Patient*'s alignment between a body and its past, Emily remarks that, "You are your history. If you cut any of it off you're an amputee" (49). While the loss of knowledge about the past can feel like losing a limb, Naomi also feels that her aunt's relentless inquiries present their own kind of surgery. "Aunt Emily," she asks, "are you a surgeon cutting at my scalp with your folders and your filing cards and your insistence on knowing all?" (178). She demands relief from the pain of this medicalized attack on the bliss of ignorance: "bring back the anaesthetist turn on the ether clamp down the gas mask bring on the chloroform when will this operation be over Aunt Em?" (178). Kogawa presents knowing and uncovering the past as an invasive medical procedure. While Emily is usually the one inflicting this kind of wound, when Naomi asks her what she thinks happened to her mother and grandmother in Japan, her aunt is startled to be asked: "It was as if my unexpected question was a sudden beam of pain that had to be extinguished immediately" (169). Pain attends the search for knowledge in *Obasan*, and the act of narration. Etymologically the words are related: the Latin word *gnārus*, "knowing," is a root for both "narrate" and "know" ("Narrate"). Storytelling is a form of knowing and a way of transmitting pain from one body to another.

Obasan frequently presents emotional connection as physical attachment. Her uncle, a devoted fisherman, never returned to the ocean after the internment, and Naomi says of him, "The sea is severed from your veins" (24). Kogawa presents the emotional loss as a physical injury. Such rupture is most pronounced in Naomi's loss of her mother. When her mother leaves for Japan to look after her own grandmother because she is ill, the child Naomi questions how her need of her mother can be supplanted by her grandmother's (64), showing the trade-offs the family members are forced to make between physical and emotional needs and connections. Naomi explains herself as a child as an offshoot from the tree of her mother's body (62) and feels disconnected for the first time as a result of her sexual abuse: "If I tell my mother about Mr. Gower, the alarm will send a tremor through our bodies and I will be torn from her. But the secret has already separated us" (62). The abuse, which has forcibly detached her from her mother, also makes her feel that her "legs are being sawn in half" (62). This feeling returns when, as an adult, she returns to the feeling she had the night of the bomb: "In the dark Slocan night, the bright light flares in my dreaming. I hear the screams and feel the mountain breaking. Your long black hair falls and falls into the chasm. My legs are sawn in half" (222). Through the repetition of this line, Kogawa aligns the pain of Naomi's mother's near destruction with the agony of her abuse and their rupture from each other. The atonement Naomi is able to find derives from her return to the idea that she is attached to her mother's body once more: "Your leg is a tree trunk and I am branch, vine, butterfly. I am joined to your limbs by right of birth, child of your flesh, leaf of your bough" (222). Emotional attachment is physical.

In this book about characters whose houses have been stolen from them, their homes also represent parts of their bodies. "This house," Obasan says, "this body. Everything old" (19), and Naomi observes that the parts and clutter of her house are part of her physical presence: "This house is now her blood and bones!" (19). This portrait of an elderly person's attachment to her dwelling should be of note for medical workers involved in geriatric care: the departure from the home can be a signal moment in the life and health of older people, and this novel offers a helpful explanation of just how physical that rupture can feel.

Wordlessness and silence represent an important source of historical injury. Early on Naomi explains that in Japanese, "The word for 'lost' also means 'dead'" (26). It is difficult for these characters, who have lost so much and so many, sometimes without knowing whether the loss has involved a death, to move beyond the obfuscation in this homonym. Naomi is not sure whether anyone ever said her father had died after his long absence. Though she remembers the moment when the news arrives, "It's possible the words are never said outright" (189). Through the distance of years, Naomi still struggles to hear her mother, but "The only sound that reaches me now is the sigh of your remembered breath, a wordless word" (221). The idea of a "wordless word" encapsulates Kogawa's many references to the unspoken and unspeakable. As an adult, Naomi's questioning about the fate of her mother is chronic but drained of hope of an answer:

> Just a glimpse of a worn-out patchwork quilt and the old question comes thudding out of the night again like a giant moth. Why did my mother not return? After all these years, I find myself wondering, but with the dullness of expecting no response.
>
> *(27)*

This question without hope of an answer recalls the opening lines of the book: "There is a silence that cannot speak. There is a silence that will not speak" (5). Kogawa's novel is an attempt to give words to that silence, without overwriting the unspeakable pain it contains.

Kogawa both expresses the unspeakable nature of the horrors suffered by Naomi's family and gives them a way to narrate and know what happened. Naomi's family only receive information about the fate of their loved ones in Nagasaki years later, through letters from Naomi's grandmother that explain their horrific injuries and losses due to the atomic bomb. Naomi's mother's face has been completely destroyed (216), and she demands that her children never be told the extent of her injuries (221). For Naomi longing for her mother, "All that is left is your word, 'Do not tell . . . '" (222). It is ironic and indicative of this novel's preoccupation with wordless words that the final words from her mother left to Naomi are an exhortation not to speak. Kogawa presents Naomi's persistent longing for her mother as an absence of writing and a desire to know. "At the age of questioning," Naomi says, "my mother disappeared. Why, I have asked ever since, did she not write? Why, I ask now, must I know?" (209). The narrative itself is an effort to come to greater knowledge of the past. At first in Japan, Naomi's mother and grandmother "were unable to talk of all the things that happened. The horror would surely die sooner, they felt, if they refused to speak" (216). But Naomi's grandmother decides to write of their experiences to her husband still in Canada because "the silence and the constancy of the nightmare had become unbearable" (216). She hopes that writing will relieve her "from the grip of the past" (216), and that "If these matters are sent away in this letter, perhaps they will depart a little from our souls" (216). The novel itself represents a similar act of hopefulness in the face of silence, the idea that narrating these horrors can relieve the pain.

The novel finally declares that silence is its own destructive injury. "Gentle Mother," the narrator writes, "we were lost together in our silences. Our wordlessness was our mutual destruction" (223). The novel connects the damage done to Naomi in her abuse and her inability to tell her mother about it to her mother's near destruction in Nagasaki and her own refusal to speak of it to her children. In a scene read by Sinéad McDermott for its revelations of Kogawa's representation of trauma and shame (158–59), Naomi recounts a recurrent dream of a doubly wounded child, injured both on her knee and her skull, and says, "The child is forever unable to speak. The child forever fears to tell" (223). She ministers to the wound, saying "I beg that the woundedness may be healed and that the limbs may learn to dance. But you stay in a black and white photograph, smiling your yasashi smile" (223). Wordlessness is part of the injury, both of the bomb, and of Naomi's abuse. *Obasan* can be read as an effort to recoup words, narrative, from an unspeakable past, to find a way to tell the story in order to heal, and to survive.

Michael Ondaatje's *The English Patient* (1992)

Given that Canadians often regard the provision of medical care as one of their defining cultural values, it's interesting that one of this country's most famous novels concerns a patient and foregrounds a character's experience of care in its title. *The English Patient* (1992) won the Booker prize and the Governor General's Award (Solecki) and has sold well over a million copies (Ratliff). In 1997, its star-studded film adaptation won nine Academy Awards including Best Picture (Bauer). Though other authors and books have enjoyed critical acclaim on a world stage, as seen for example with Alice Munro's 2012 Nobel Prize and Margaret Atwood's ongoing celebration for and adaptations of *The Handmaid's Tale* (1985) (see Wells-Lassagne and McMahon), the watershed moment of *The English Patient*'s popularity must be regarded as a high point of the international success of Canadian literature.

In Ondaatje's novel, four characters displaced by WWII find refuge in a bombed Italian villa that had housed German soldiers and then an Allied infirmary (12–13). Only one patient remains, an Englishman burned beyond recognition, along with a young nurse, Hana, who abandoned her post to stay with him when all the other medical workers left. They are joined by Kip, a Sikh sapper, or bomb defuser, from India with whom she has a romance, and Caravaggio, a Canadian thief whom she knew in Toronto (47). While the characters at first believe the patient's account of his identity, Caravaggio uncovers the truth of his Hungarian nationality and his collaboration with the Nazis, concluding, in the key irony of this book concerned with irony, that "the English patient is not English" (163).

The patient's injuries are near total, as he clings to life without skin, identity, or motion, and the novel explores the recuperation of history from such an all-but-destroyed person. Ondaatje pushes the patient's incapacity to this extreme to question what happens to character when all that's left of a body is memory and to offer an allegory of history itself lying in ashes. We can connect Ondaatje's dual focus on the scene of medical ministration and the writing of the past through the idea of the patient history. Taking a medical history is a component of the diagnostic process, but storytelling and history in a broad sense also diagnose: they recount the past to explain its result. In English the word "patient" implies a person who is subject to a medical system of care, but also the idea of patience, acceptant waiting, though it is derived from "pati," the Latin word for suffering ("Patient"). While the patient's Englishness is always in question and eventually disproven, readers should also be alive to whether he is in fact patient, what he is or was waiting for, and, if he is subject to a medical system, whose it is. The answers to these questions change throughout the book, signalling the ironic complexities Ondaatje develops to explore human psyches through the metaphor of a shifting desert.

In examining Ondaatje's postmodern depiction of injury, I begin by discussing the gendered stakes of caring in this novel, before addressing the exchange of morphine for narrative and the addictions of each, followed by an account of how the patient's body represents a physical source of history, like a book.

Nursing, Gender, and Care

One way to read this war novel that transpires after a war has ended, and that was published nearly fifty years later, is as dramatizing a scene of care to engage belated, uncaring readers. We can read the shell-shocked nurse's story as directed at readers who, detached from the history, might themselves be struggling to care about the now-distant crisis of World War II.

The novel questions how and why people care, for the injured, but also about the past.

The English Patient is often taught as an example of literary postmodernism because of its fragmented style, but, like another major postmodern work, Toni Morrison's *Beloved* (1987), it can also be classed as a historical novel. Historical fiction often projects the hero's journey as a stand-in for the cultural progress of a nation, as the theorist Georg Lukács discussed previously suggests. Reading Ondaatje's novel through this lens invites a view of the journeying Canadian war nurse, Hana, as one such national representative. The intensity of the regard Ondaatje lavishes on her altruistic care could be put in conversation with notions of the Canadian value placed on publicly funded healthcare, so that the novel could be read for its articulation of a core Canadian ethos, its creation of a World War II myth to explain subsequent decades of public policy.

The book layers therapeutic relationships throughout its pages, with the patient at the centre of a multiplicity of medicinal, one-to-one connections radiating outward. Vikki Visvis considers the extent to which the novel reflects psychoanalytic notions of the talking cure, a salient context especially given that Ondaatje himself has described the novel as "a book about very tentative healing among a group of people" (qtd. in Visvis 90). While the nurse Hana is the patient's primary caregiver, Caravaggio takes on a version of that role as his dealer, Kip himself becomes a doctor years after the main events of the novel (299), and the patient's mind persistently wanders back to the desert doctor who ministered to him from his vast collection of bottles (10). Checking on her patient, Hana assumes that in sleep his mind is back in the desert with a healer who holds salves in a "bowl made with the joined soles of his feet" (35). This lost desert doctor is the original model for the relations of care on which the patient has come to rely. A man burned almost into oblivion, he remains dependent on versions of this now-essential doctor–patient relationship.

The story begins partly in a nurse's failure to do her job: she refuses the order to leave the villa to lavish all her care on one last patient. Margaret McAllister reads the novel as an allegory for the nurse as "wounded healer," while James Metcalf writes of using this novel to teach best practices to nursing students, but Ondaatje's story can also be read as a nurse's refusal of the norms of her profession. Ministering to a single patient with this extreme level of care was not in the regular workflow of a war nurse, who would normally have had to give the minimum attention to more patients than her shift could accommodate (Harris 72, see also Brooks and Hallet). By scrutinizing Hana's idiosyncratic response to her patient, Ondaatje's book questions how much one person can care, and when care ends.

The book constructs the nurse's professional refusal as a result of her own injuries. When "The burned man noticed the young nurse," he "knew she was more patient than nurse" (96). Even caregivers can need care and can suffer from pathologies. Though she's not physically injured, she is said to be suffering from "Partial shell shock probably" (28). Ondaatje writes that "Nurses too became shell-shocked from the dying around them" (41) or would crack "the way Hana broke" when she learned of her father's death (41). Her loss of a pregnancy (82–85) also contributes to her accumulation of sorrow, and her experiences result in her refusal to care under the system of her employment. After the war, Ondaatje writes, she would not follow orders but only her own rules, and "would care only for the burned patient" (14). Though caring is the role of a nurse, ironically, the nurse's injury is evident in her failure to stop caring for a patient. The disruption to her usual role as a nurse starts this story and is caused by her own illness.

Ondaatje emphasizes the refusal of both patient and nurse to conform to the decrees of the medical system under which they had been living. They "had insisted on remaining behind when the other nurses and patients moved to a safer location in the south" (13), they "had refused to leave" (28), and now "he is her last patient in the Villa San Girolamo, their war over, both of them refusing to return with the others to the safety of the Pisa hospitals" (41). This repetition emphasizes how their failure to depart was not an accident of timing, or a practical response to the patient's incapacity, but, for both of them, it was a refusal, a far more considered and deliberate response. Both are refusing to continue operating in the prior system ordering their lives.

Even beyond her refusal of the order of her medical superiors to abandon him in favour of the care of others more likely to survive, the version of medical care Hana pursues with the patient is unusual. She climbs into his bed to warm him (5), bites pits from plums for him (4, 45), and, like lovers, their intimacy occurs beyond words, as "she blows cool air onto his neck, and he mutters" (4). Ondaatje revels in exploring new textures for the structure of their unusual nurse–patient relationship, suggesting for example that "She was living like a vagrant, while elsewhere the English patient reposed in his bed like a king" (14). Both are playing medical roles that can shift with a label.

Ondaatje offers a historical illustration of the burdens of care facing war nurses like Hana and a portrait of the expectations of their profession. Offering to help Caravaggio, Hana proclaims, "I can get you off the morphine, you know. I'm a good nurse" (266). Yet for Hana, war has altered what it means to be a "good nurse," whether the label implies professional excellence, or a strong moral compass. Ondaatje recounts her education and entry into the system, explaining how "She herself had been trained at Women's College Hospital" in Toronto and then joined the war effort overseas in 1943 (49). The job of nursing requires an emotional response, empathy with patients, that war complicates by throwing forward too many patients, too many to care for. The intense empathy of nursing is represented in how Hana literally walks in the shoes of a dead patient (50). Yet the patient is simply dead and unknown, and, since in taking his shoes "she ignored all rules" (50), the move could be regarded as theft, showing the shifting and often futile results of the nurse's empathy. Hana's trouble is that although she has trained in a profession of care, she is no longer able to follow rules for caring.

The war nurse discovers that the only way to manage the overwhelming emotional burden of nursing war casualties is to regard caring as something that ends. Hana learns that "Caring was brief. There was a contract only until death" (51). Though at first she could feel a tenderness towards soldiers she didn't know, a kind of "tenderness to the self" (49), later the lack of prevailing reason and order hardens her towards both herself and her patients (50). "Throughout the war," Ondaatje writes, "with all of her worst patients, she survived by keeping a coldness hidden in her role as a nurse" (48). Working as a nurse meant that "she secretly pulled her personal self back," a retrenchment common to so many of her colleagues in nursing, who "had turned into emotionally disturbed handmaidens of the war" (178). The labour of war nursing obstructs the women's ability to care beyond professional requirements.

Indeed, as the book progresses, it becomes clear that Hana's intense care for the patient replaces the care she wishes she could have offered her father as he died. Like the English patient, her father was also terribly burned, and died of his injuries (295). Before the news of his death, "She feared the day she would remove blood from a patient's face and discover her father" (50). Each of her charges is a potential stand-in for her father, just as the English patient too becomes. She wonders if her father was "nursed by a stranger" (90) before he died, and laments that she wasn't with him, because she says, "I know a lot about burning," and "He was a burned man and I was a nurse and I could have nursed him" (296). Here we see the return of the roles of "burned man" and "nurse" that Hana has used to organize her unusual relationship with the English patient. Her relentless care for him is an attempt to make good her knowledge of burns, as a form of atonement for the care she couldn't give her father. Hana insists that "Till the nuns reclaimed it she would sit in this villa with the Englishman" (52), raising the question of what she might do with his body, and whether her commitment to his burned shell would endure beyond death, in a gruesome possibility reminiscent of William Faulkner's short story "A Rose for

Emily" (1930). Only when it emerges that the English patient is a stand-in for her father does her relentless care for him make sense.

In discussing Hana's uneasy relationship with the profession of nursing, it's important to consider how the historical feminization of the role dovetails with a potential critique of gender roles in this novel. As is often the case in the profession of nursing itself, caring in this book is offloaded to women. Even as she is persistently sexualized by the men around her, the main female character is always administering care to them. Recalling the historic feminization of nursing, Caravaggio explains, in answer to the question of who cut off his thumbs, that "They found a woman to do it" (55). The subjugation of women in nursing roles, and the shunting of the horrors of war to their laps, gives force to Hana's anger in claiming that "Every damn general should have had my job" (84). The authority for war is assigned to men, while its pain and messes are given over to women. The fact that in later life Kip becomes a doctor (299) shows how the gendered hierarchy between the roles of doctor and nurse is repeated between these characters. Even her physical affection for Kip is presented as an offering in parallel to her ministrations to the other two men in the villa, since he "does not need or want the drug in a needle she could slide into his arm, as Caravaggio does, or those ointments of desert invention the Englishman craves" (126). Ondaatje aligns her romance with Kip as an extension of her role as a nurse, writing that it was "only a step past" the physical comforts she'd offered dying patients (126). It could be argued that Ondaatje frames the relationship in this way, as a kind of alternative act of nursing, to extend his construction of Hana's pathological relationship to her profession due to shell shock. For twenty-first century readers, however, this construction of romantic love as an extension of workplace exigencies may mark the age of Ondaatje's novel, and its composition in a time defined by different gender politics.

Morphine, Theft, and Narrative

Alongside care, Ondaatje's book also questions the methods, goals, and artefacts of history. The two greatest fetishes of this narrative, books and morphine, promise conduits to a sense of the past that can only endure in fragments. Drug addiction and the theft and doling out of medications both to ease pain and promote storytelling are key components of this story. Hana's power is in her "little box of medical supplies" (14), and the stash of "codeine tablets, as well as the morphine" that she "salted away" when the other nurses left (42). She professes to "know death now" (83), but this dark knowledge also includes the role of morphine: she says, of soldiers at the end of life, "I know how to divert them from agony. When to give the quick jolt of morphine in a major vein" (84). Dying in these moments sometimes involves the medication of a nurse, throwing into question the role of caregiver and the extent to which the morphine speeds death.

Both the English patient and Caravaggio are dependent on morphine. Playing upon his frequent use of the idea of ruin, Ondaatje gives an origin story for Caravaggio's addiction when introducing him in the convalescent hospital, writing that he was "in near ruins when he was brought in and given regular doses of morphine for the pain in his hands" (27). For the English patient, morphine both relieves pain and offers him a kind of travel both in time and space. As Hana medicates him, "He rides the boat of morphine. It races in him, imploding time and geography the way maps compress the world onto a two-dimensional sheet of paper" (160). Whereas the patient needs others to inject him, Caravaggio manages his dependence through theft. Stolen morphine is the currency of his relationship with Hana. Whereas she pilfered her morphine from the departing medical team, Caravaggio frequently steals from her stash. He "had sniffed out her medical supplies within hours of his arrival" (166), and steals a great deal of morphine, gorging on it (166). She hides morphine in rooms other than the English patient's so Caravaggio doesn't bother him (125), while Caravaggio often goes "rifling through her medicine chest" before "injecting the morphine quickly into himself" (85). Their various uses for and dependencies on morphine draw the characters into action and potential conflict with each other.

Of all the characters, Caravaggio is most preoccupied with the drug, and most certain that he can use it to achieve his goals, namely, of forcing the truth from the patient. He injects the patient with morphine to extract his story: Caravaggio gets the patient talking "because I gave him an extra dose of morphine" (163), and he says, "I'd like to talk with him some more. With some morphine in him" (166). Hearing a patient's story is normally the precursor to the administration of medicine, not the result. It is significant that it is a thief who thus corrupts the role of prescriber, so that a figure who normally steals becomes a giver, to pilfer the patient's story. Caravaggio even invokes medical innovation to serve his goals: "I'll cook up a Brompton cocktail," he suggests. "Morphine and alcohol. They invented it at Brompton Hospital in London for their cancer patients" (166). Once more we see classic motives for medicine being invoked and inverted, as Caravaggio professes to want to use a concoction against pain to produce narrative. He promises Hana, "I won't damage him. The morphine and alcohol will take away the pain" (166). The pain in question here could be from the burns, or the anguish of telling his harrowing story. As Caravaggio administers the drug to advance the patient's tale, Ondaatje adds notes regarding the dosage amounts and schedule as though compiling a medical file: "3 CC's Brompton cocktail. 3:00 p.m." (167). The insertion aligns the taking of a medical history, the telling of a personal story while intoxicated, and the work of fiction. Throughout this book, such moments that might seem to reflect "standard" scenes of medical care are in fact distortions that show the complex shifts in morality of a world in crisis.

Ondaatje develops a direct connection between Caravaggio's delivery of morphine and the patient's storytelling. During the patient's narration, Caravaggio "stays alongside him reordering the events" (248). "When the burnt man slows down, or when Caravaggio feels he's not catching everything," Ondaatje writes, "he picks up the syringe from the kidney-shaped enamel tin, breaks the glass tip off an ampoule with the pressure of a knuckle and loads it" (247). Caravaggio medicates the patient to keep his story going. "Each swallow of morphine by the body opens a further door," Ondaatje writes, one that returns the patient to the cave, or his lover's body (247). In a kind of opium den scene, Caravaggio and the patient take morphine together as they move more deeply into the story (243). The patient says "I have come to love the tap of your fingernail on the syringe, Caravaggio" (238). With their shared world of addiction and shared enthrallment with the patient's story, their intimacy—and co-dependence—becomes more intense. Desperate to learn the truth, Caravaggio is held captive by the suspense of the patient's tale, while the patient uses his narrative to control his access to morphine. Stopping in midstream, he silently demands another tablet with an outstretched hand before continuing (174). Morphine fuels the story, and narrative is the drug the patient exchanges for morphine.

Yet despite his own choice to administer the medication to hear the patient's story, Caravaggio soon feels trapped by the addictive basis of the relationship. He knows "he must get out of this desert, its architecture of morphine" (251). His power over the situation has shifted, even as the patient needles him, demanding that "You must talk to me, Caravaggio. Or am I just a book? Something to be read, some creature to be tempted out of a loch and shot full of morphine" (253). The patient's story has become one of Caravaggio's addictions, one that he also spurs with morphine, and that likewise brings him into a toxic state from which he dreams of escape (251). Caravaggio sees his administration of morphine to the patient as a kind of abuse for his own purposes of learning the real story, and so is surprised to recognize that the patient "has used him and the morphine to return to his own world" (251). Addictive drugs throw into question who is a user and who is being used.

In Caravaggio's perverse therapy there is the hint that telling his story could be a part of the patient's pain relief, but it becomes clear that this relation is not direct. Despite the implication that narrative itself could relieve pain, in fact, the patient trades his story for his painkilling drug of choice. Who plays the role of care provider keeps shifting throughout this book, while the patient's storytelling can be read either as his own careful drug deal, in which he doles out enough scraps of narrative to keep Caravaggio's morphine coming, or as Caravaggio's own abusive theft of the patient's story.

History, Books, and Bodies

In the logic of Ondaatje's book, a burned person is a burned history, and the patient's body itself is a proxy for the ruins of civilization, from which a new world order must grow after World War II. Caravaggio, as he tries to squeeze narrative out of the patient by squeezing morphine in, describes the patient's stories as his "histories" (107). As the patient "speaks sometimes in the first person, sometimes in the third person" (247), the novel continuously rewrites the viewpoint from which his history is expressed, just as the roles of patient and caregiver frequently shift. Whose history is getting resurrected and why is always in question. Ondaatje's alignment between the resurrection of the past and a traumatized body contributes to how the novel exemplifies Linda Hutcheon's notion of historiographic metafiction (see McVey). The book processes the aftermath of war through other dangerous extremes, from the risks of desert exploration to the often-terminal dangers of bomb diffusion and morphine addiction. In its belated account of this aftermath, the novel fetishizes the notion of history and locates it in material objects, books, and bodies. Their preservation, even in ruins, promises to preserve the past itself.

Through this reading, the postmodern stakes of Ondaatje's historical novel become clear. The patient's body can be read as a burned yet nevertheless readable book. This novel about storytelling aligns books and bodies like other influential postmodern works from the 1990s, including Peter Greenaway's *The Pillow Book* (1996), and Jeanette Winterson's *Written on the Body* (1992), published the same year as *The English Patient.* Coalescing the metafictional tendencies of this work, the burned body at the heart of Ondaatje's novel symbolizes his historical novel itself, as the story questions the possibility of capturing narrative about the past from the bonfire of time.

Ondaatje's book is itself a compendium of excerpts from other histories and uses fiction to question the possibility of an unfragmented story, with the burned patient's body indicating a ravaged sense of time. The idea of the desert and his copy of Herodotus' *Histories* both define the patient's character and localize a notion of history. The desert, the patient's major obsession, represents the irresistible enigma of the past. The patient describes his mapping work there as the "slow unearthing of history in the desert" (241), which the war interrupts. In the desert water comes and goes in "Sporadic appearances and disappearances, like legends and rumours through history" (141). The copy of Herodotus, besides being a history book itself, also contains the patient's own accumulation of personal records and notes (16). Described as "his holy book" (294), it is "the book he had somehow managed to carry with him out of the fire" (94). He is someone who "speaks in fragments" (96) and fills "his 1890 edition of Herodotus' *Histories*" with "other fragments—maps, diary entries, writings in many languages, paragraphs cut out of other books. All that is missing is his own name" (96). The book contains his identity, as much as his body does. He tells Katharine he needs to keep his Herodotus with him, for it is "more a commonplace book" in which he keeps his notes (231). He carries the book as a kind of talisman (237), often asks for it or picks it up to read while in the villa (118, 247), explaining that "What you find in him are cul-de-sacs within the sweep of history" (119). Referencing Hutcheon's discussions of Ondaatje's postmodernism, Vernon Provencal interprets how the copy of Herodotus illustrates an ambivalence towards history in the novel. Just as the patient's notes fill his Herodotus, Hana writes a diary in *The Last of the Mohicans* (61), suggesting that in this postwar world, new history must be written into old books. Writing their stories into ancient volumes gives these characters a way to move forward from their cataclysms.

Romantic love represents an alternative form of history that connects the past of lovers through their bodies. The patient describes his romance with Katharine as the "story of how I fell in love with a woman, who read me a specific story from Herodotus" (233). He glues notes on their affair "into sections of *The Histories* that recorded wars that were of no interest to him" (172). "When we meet those we fall in love with," the patient says, "there is an aspect of our spirit that is historian" (259). When Hana spends time with Kip in his tent, "they are never sure what will occur, whose fraction of past will emerge" (270). The patient contrasts this historical aspect of romance with the details noted in official accounts of the past, saying that their adultery will not appear "in the minutes of the Geographical Society" or those "detailed reports which chartered every knoll and every incident of history" (145). Their romance is so linked in his mind to his own work of writing that he cannot stop thinking about her while he writes his book:

> I was unable to remove her body from the page. I wished to dedicate the monograph to her, to her voice, to her body that I imagined rose white out of a bed like a long bow, but it was a book I dedicated to a king.
> *(235)*

Katharine's body itself becomes central to the book he writes, just as the patient's own burned body is the crucial object of Ondaatje's. The patient identifies as a jackal, in whose "jaws are pieces of the past he delivers to you" (259), and he says, "I wish for all this to be marked on my body when I am dead" (261). The past is contained in and written on the body.

The more common physical containers of history, however, are books, which were targets of arson in Nazi Germany (see Rose). The patient's observation that "We are communal histories, communal books" (261) makes explicit this connection between personhood, history, and books, and helps explain why the novel foregrounds experiences of reading and the materiality of texts. The overt preoccupation with books as objects in Ondaatje's text contributes to his study of whether and how the past can be physically preserved. The object of the book has long been essential to the transmission of history as well as literature, and in this novel about injury and history, books stand in for the frailties of human bodies and memory.

Ruined books, bodies, and buildings analogize history in this text that keeps returning to acts of reading. The patient, whose room is stacked with books (93), gives lessons on how to read (94). Hana reads to him "from whatever book she is able to find in the library downstairs" (5), is often to be found with a book herself (282), as she "fell upon books as the only door out of her cell" (7). She keeps reading to him even after he's asleep, so the stories "had gaps of plot" that Ondaatje compares to storm-damaged roads, locust-eaten tapestries, and bombed murals (7). This description of a story in ruins matches their nearly destroyed villa (7), where even the library is open to rain, and its books get wet (8). The matter-of-fact response to destroyed books results from a practical response to the destruction all around. The staircase is missing some levels, so Hana repairs it by nailing books from the library into new steps (13). In this story of books as building materials, Ondaatje develops a spatial analogy for narrative, which transpires in his book as a kind of reconstruction. Ruined books become materials for patching up a ruined house for a body in ruins who tells a fragmented history of ruin. Ondaatje here layers ruin upon ruin to illustrate the historical extremity of these characters' lives and encounters with time. All their buildings have been bombed and are ruins, and so are their stories, the histories, like the patient's body itself.

The novel consistently foregrounds the materiality of communication in letters as well as books, as pages can be burned like bodies. The patient speaks of Kipling as "a writer who used pen and ink" (94), while Hana dwells on the materiality of her stepmother's letters, which she imagines being written in a notebook on a windy Georgian Bay shore (91). The lovers are "intimate like two pages of a closed book" (155), while Hana revels in the physicality of books, their "spines" (221), and "the smell of them, even the sound of the crack if you open them too fast, as if breaking some minute unseen series of bones" (222). Recalling the patient's own view of Katharine's body in his book, the idea of bones in books furthers Ondaatje's analogy between bodies and history. Books as objects are so essential to human continuance that the patient even replaces his material fetish object of morphine with a book: "ignoring the tablet that brings painlessness" (298), he "touches his book" and "nothing else moves in the room" (298). The patient is "a person who if left alone in someone's home walks to the bookcase, pulls down a volume and inhales it. So history enters us" (18). The consumption of information in books is a way of integrating history with the body.

In the context of Ondaatje's preoccupation with the physicality of history, romance represents an inflection point between bodies and their pasts. Rather than equating physical love with pleasure, this story presents romance as pain and injury. The patient makes the gruesome observation that "you can make love to a woman with a broken arm, or a woman with a fever" (170), and the lovers taste each other's blood (170), and she licks his tears (157). Their relationship consists of "A list of wounds" (153), as the patient catalogues the physical injuries Katharine gives him (153), claiming that "He has been disassembled by her" (155). As they try to end their affair, she bangs her head on a gatepost as they leave each other (158) in a moment that recalls Emily Brontë's Heathcliff banging his head against a tree out of romantic frustration and grief (204). The pain of injuries offers a proxy for the turbulence of love. As Kip's mind returns to his time at the villa at the end of the novel, he reflects that perhaps his reminiscing is due to "the chemical burn on the arm of the girl he treated today" (300). Injury unlocks memory, while doctor–patient interactions provoke storytelling for both parties. Kip, the bomb defuser, whose role implies another ethics of care by putting himself in harm's way to protect the lives of others, cracks at news of the bomb to end all bombs and detaches himself from the social world in which he's become involved. In his rage he blames the English patient, as though he were English, shouting "Was it just ships that gave you such power? Was it, as my brother said, because you had the histories and printing presses?" (283). "Having" history is itself presented as a kind of political domination. As news of the bomb spreads Ondaatje describes it as "A terrible event emerging out of the short wave. A new war. The death of a civilization" (286). Histories die with their civilizations. In the aftermath of this apocalypse, new histories will be written, and new fictions.

This circling of the meaning of history relates to Ondaatje's presentation of the novel itself as historical fiction. The work's self-conscious and metafictive quality seems to deconstruct its own style as an extension of its theme. In this sense, while the characters pursue a fragmentary sense of history, the fiction presents itself as another partial, and therefore possibly more trenchant, version of the past. Ondaatje's prose itself sometimes slips into a historical register to advance its story from the screen of a distant and neutral perspective (95), or it includes fragments of historical reportage (134). The author quotes from Tacitus' *Annals* as a book that begins with an "assurance of order," whereas, he writes, "novels commenced with hesitation or chaos" (93). Ondaatje puts fiction forward as a disordered, and possibly therefore more truthful, counterpart to written history. A quintessential text for understanding the fragmentations of postmodern literary style, this work presents itself as another commonplace book alongside the patient's precious copy of Herodotus. Like the patient's own deconstructed body and his partial fragmentary storytelling, *The English Patient* exists as a scrapbook that puts the sutured structure of its narrative on display. As his characters make their lives in this story that is itself as split up as the bombed nunnery in which they take shelter, Ondaatje's observation that "They were protected by the simple fact that the villa seemed a ruin" (14) reflects the workings of his own novel. Ondaatje's book uses the fragmenting affordances of postmodern style to explore what salvation characters can find in the ruins war has made of their lives and their sense of history.

Ironies accumulate in this book, from the Englishman who is not English, to the nurse who refuses both to nurse and to stop nursing, to the villa's shelter that is a ruin. One more irony for this book about irony and the afterlives of books and people concerns the Egyptian desert cave covered in ancient paintings of swimming where the patient leaves Katharine (169). Though the desert scenes in Anthony Minghella's film adaptation of the novel were shot in Tunisia, the real "Cave of Swimmers" became overrun after the movie increased its fame and the subsequent arrival of GPS technology helped tourists find it, leading to efforts to mitigate negative impacts on its drawings (see Riemer and Kuper). The site encapsulates persistent ironies of the desert in the novel, since, the English patient explains, "In Wadi Sura I saw caves whose walls were covered with paintings of swimmers" (18). The caves themselves represent a trajectory of climate change, so that a site once known for swimmable waters is now in the heart of the desert. These swimmers may be depicted in an afterlife, however, adding to the ghostliness of this multilayered symbol. Given the impact of *The English Patient*'s fame on this site, this book about the destruction of the past should also be read for its own inadvertent degradation of history: Ondaatje's novel about injury to the past has caused its own.

In this anecdote lies a parable for how a book can contribute to the human factors causing environmental desecration and the sometimes-pathological outcomes of storytelling. Stories themselves can cause injury and harm. As much as *The English Patient* is a book about recuperating history from a destroyed body, it has contributed to both the degradation—and now, as a result, the preservation—of far older stories painted onto the cave walls of Wadi Sura.

Shani Mootoo's *Cereus Blooms at Night* (1996)

Amid this array of postmodern novels that concern storytelling relationships between the injured and their caregivers, nurses in particular, Shani Mootoo's *Cereus Blooms at Night* (1996) represents an important document. Though now rarely mentioned in popular discourse, the novel has sparked a rich and ongoing breadth of scholarly discussion, with dozens of critical articles exploring, for example, the politics and healing of sexual hybridity in the novel (Pirbhai), its representations of trans embodiments (Ku), the empowerments of care and disability (Nielsen), and its depiction of mental illness (Cvetkovich 140–55; Mardorossian).

In the novel, set on a fictional Caribbean island called Lantanacamara, the care of Miss Mala Ramchandin, a psychiatric patient troubled by a history of sexual abuse, comes under the care of Tyler, an assigned-male but gender-fluid orderly who is gradually permitted to take on the role of her nurse. Mootoo's 2008 essay, "On Becoming an Indian Starboy," offers important context for the gender complexity in this novel, but Mootoo does not specify new pronouns for Tyler other than masculine, so I follow most scholars in using he/him pronouns to refer to this character. Nevertheless, it's worth observing that his status as a first-person narrator largely keeps Mootoo from needing to use pronouns to refer to him. Mootoo presents the novel as Tyler's effort to transcribe Mala's story for the benefit of her long-lost sister. Like the other books considered in this chapter, the novel regards narrative as a product of the exchange between damaged patients and their caregivers.

Tyler's model of nursing contends with the restrictive gendering of the profession, while engaging with its uniforms. "I was, after all," he says, "the only Lantanacamaran man ever to have trained in the profession of nursing" (6). He dresses for the role of nurse (6), but at first is only put to work cleaning (6). Because Miss Ramchandin is difficult, and no one else wants to go by her room, Tyler explains that her "care was therefore left in my hands, and I was finally able to employ my nursing skills" (13). A relation of care thus grows between the difficult patient and the problem nurse, who defies the gender roles of nursing. Though Tyler at one point is to be taken off her care, she resists by dismantling and rearranging her room (97–99), so he "got to keep [his] full-time job caring for Miss Ramchandin" (99). She's supposed to be bound, but Tyler loosens her straps

(12), and she steals a female nurse's uniform for him (75). Tyler's moves toward expressing a different gender identity happen partly through adopting the costumes of nursing. He finds himself "becoming protective of her" (24), and is credited with the improvement in her demeanour, but he resists the praise, "knowing the change in Miss Ramchandin was only a result of humane treatment" (97). The healing afforded by good nursing, which Tyler describes simply as "humane," is here discounted, but his performance of the model nurse delivers the real deal.

The textured relationship between the nurse and his charge informs the structure of the text itself. Tyler explains that he felt driven to look after Miss Ramchandin "because I felt an empathy for her clenched fists, defiant stare, pursed lips and deep, slow, calculated breathing—an empathy that words alone cannot describe" (19). While this assertion underscores the intimacy between caregivers and their patients, the novel itself, Tyler's narrative about Miss Ramchandin, seems to be his response to this failure of language to express his compassion for her. The novel is his effort to fill in this particular gap with words after all.

Always pulling at the status and motives of Tyler's story is the question of his own gender identity and sexuality. He experiences desire towards men (70, 102), and flirts with a male doctor: "That the doctor's presence made me blush is not important to this story, but to ignore how alive and frisky I felt in his presence would be to deny the part of me that hopes for freedom" (22). Tyler describes himself as "neither properly man nor woman but some in-between, unnamed thing" (71). His wish to shake what he calls his "perversion" leads to an interest in the "perverse," which the Ramchandins' sad family story of incest seems to represent (47–48). The recurrent tension between Tyler's wish to be free—out and accepted—and his role as Miss Ramchandin's biographer gives the text a compelling undercurrent. He makes the link between his sexuality and his ability to tell her story explicit, describing

> the positions I was in that enabled me to gain the full story. For there were two: one, a shared queerness with Miss Ramchandin, which gave rise to the other, my proximity to the very Ramchandin Nana herself had known of.
>
> *(48)*

Mootoo continuously circles the question of whether and how Tyler's own sexual and gender identity "matters" to this story.

By times Tyler's own story offers to break through to dominate the narrative, overcoming its biographical focus on Miss Ramchandin, but he consistently steps back to the role of narrator alone. Rather than giving in to the temptation to narrate his long experience with homophobic microaggressions, he says, "I must be strict with myself and stay with my intention to relate Mala Ramchandin's story" (15). He opens the second part of the book by claiming that "You will hear little more of me" (105). Mootoo sets up the text as Tyler's appeal to Miss Ramchandin's sister to visit her sibling (3). In his effort to learn and document his patient's story, he enjoys the irony that "for all the scant attention paid my presence, I am the one who ended up knowing the truth, the whole truth, every significant *and* insignificant bit of it" (6–7). He takes a certain pride in being the "one who is putting it all to good use by recording it here" (7) in case it might compel Miss Ramchandin's sister to visit. With the help of some visitors from her past, Tyler explains, "I was able to fill in gaps and make sense of things she mumbled" (102). Tyler is as involved with Miss Ramchandin as her biographer and historian as much as her nurse. At times Tyler wonders whether, in a parallel for the work of the novelist, his effort veers into transcribing what might be fantasy or nonsense: "As much as I had learned not to discount her mental fitness, I must admit there were times when I believed her words were fanciful imaginings. I wrote everything down though, just in case" (102). Tyler's version of nursing involves transcription, not simply of medical notes and medication schedules, but Miss Ramchandin's life story.

Though he works as a nurse, Tyler's greatest labour is as a writer. He is presented as a constantly diarizing presence, always in the act of transcribing events as they happen like the heroines of Samuel Richardson's epistolary novels, and also reconstructing others' stories about the past. Tyler is ostensibly writing this narrative to present it to Miss Ramchandin's lost sister as an enticement for her to visit, a premise maintained until the final page (249). Yet at the end of the novel it emerges that Asha herself has written a collection of unanswered letters to her sister (243) and has also become a nurse (245). Tyler and Asha thus mirror each other as writing caregivers. Readers should consider what purpose might be served by this note-taking, and what motives or obsessions might compel it. Mootoo's novel raises the question of why caregivers might write down anything beyond the required measurements and dosages that make up the dull progress of sick days. An impulse to document and preserve attends sick and injured bodies and is thus readily available to their caregivers—but such patients also give narrators something to talk about, trouble to relate. The ill patient presents the caregiver inclined to storytelling with an opportunity. In that light we should question whether Tyler is using the pretence of conveying Miss Ramchandin's story for the opportunity to tell his own, a perspective that clarifies the persistent eruptions of Tyler's autobiographical impulse. Telling Miss Ramchandin's story lets Tyler tell his.

As Mootoo's novel illustrates, the storytelling caregiver offers social rehabilitation and advocacy to their patients, a chance of historical preservation and a point of access between the inarticulacy of suffering and the procedures of the hospital and broader social world.

Conclusion

Each of these novels reveals an effort to recoup a narrative of the past, a history, from the aftermath of disastrous injury. The almost terminally injured body that still speaks offers a parable for the postmodern idea that narrating atrocity means gathering the fragments of a scattered archive. The shredded body analogizes a history sifted out from ashes: the talking patient with a fully bandaged face represents the inevitability of trying to speak of disaster, despite its world-ending ruptures.

Caregivers in fiction frequently stand as the final witnesses to the truth of atrocities, and they must tell their patients' stories or risk letting them go forever unheard. This relation mirrors usual notions of the taking of medical history, where patients disclose their narratives so caregivers can diagnose. Here medical professionals tell their patients' stories to keep them from falling to silence with their charges' deaths. The idea of the storytelling health worker has long and widespread currency in Canada, but also abroad, with Albert Camus's *The Plague* (1947) standing as a classic example. If the trouble or conflict of the story is an injury or illness, the caregiver, as the one positioned to watch its progress, can offer authors an ideal narrator, at once professionally neutral and deeply engaged in the problem at hand.

The books discussed in this chapter often allegorize compassion as the loosening of ties. In *The English Patient*, the ties are the bandages the patient must have applied and reapplied: in one so grievously injured, the body itself is no longer a conduit to freedom. The only release the patient can hope for beyond telling his story, having it carried out of the fire like his copy of Herodotus, is an ultimate liberation from pain in death. Again and again, *The English Patient* accomplishes this deepening and reinvention of familiar tropes, which is why, in the landscape of Canadian fiction about physical trauma, this novel has proven such a lastingly arresting book.

Works Cited

Al-Rawi, Ahmed, and Kiana Zemenchik. "Tiktoking COVID-19 with Frontline Workers." *Digital Health*, vol. 9, Jan. 2023, pp. 1–8.

Bauer, Pat. "The English Patient." *Encyclopedia Britannica*, 25 Jun. 2024, www.britannica.com/topic/The-English-Patient-film-by-Minghella. Accessed 15 July 2024.

Bergen, David. *The Time in Between*. McClelland & Stewart, 2005.
Brontë, Emily. *Wuthering Heights*. 1847. Penguin, 1965.
Brooks, Jane, and Christine E. Hallett, editors. *One Hundred Years of Wartime Nursing Practices, 1854–1953*. Manchester UP, 2015.
Brydon, Diana. "Obasan: Joy Kogawa's 'Lament for a Nation'." *Kunapipi*, vol. 16, no. 1, 1994, pp. 465–70.
Caruth, Cathy. *Unclaimed Experience: Trauma, Narrative, and History*. 1996. Johns Hopkins UP, 2016.
Cvetkovich, Ann. *An Archive of Feelings: Trauma, Sexuality, and Lesbian Public Cultures*. Duke UP, 2003.
Facundo, A. C. *Oscillations of Literary Theory: The Paranoid Imperative and Queer Reparative*. SUNY, 2016.
Findley, Timothy. *The Wars*. 1977. Penguin, 2017.
Ford, Julian D., et al. "Temporal Trends in Health Worker Social Media Communication during the COVID-19 Pandemic." *Research in Nursing & Health*, vol. 45, no. 6, Dec. 2022, pp. 636–51.
Frank, Arthur W. *The Wounded Storyteller*. U of Chicago P, 1995.
Greenaway, Peter. *The Pillow Book*. Dis Voir, 1995.
Grenier, Stéphane, and Adam Montgomery. *After the War: Surviving PTSD and Changing Mental Health Culture*. U of Regina P, 2018.
Harris, Kirsty. "'All for the Boys': The Nurse-Patient Relationship of Australian Army Nurses in the First World War." *First World War Nursing: New Perspectives*, edited by Alison S. Fell and Christine E. Hallett, Routledge, 2013, pp. 71–87.
Hutcheon, Linda. *The Canadian Postmodern*. Oxford UP, 1988.
Hutcheon, Linda. *A Poetics of Postmodernism: History, Theory, Fiction*. Routledge, 1988.
Kogawa, Joy. *Obasan*. 1981. Penguin, 2006.
Kruger, Steven F. *AIDS Narratives: Gender and Sexuality, Fiction and Science*. Garland, 1996.
Ku, Chung-Hao. "Trans Bodies and Embodiments in Shani Mootoo's *Cereus Blooms at Night*." *Twentieth-Century Literature*, vol. 69, no. 1, Mar. 2023, pp. 83–104.
Lee, Kwang Chear, et al. "History of Burns: The Past, Present and the Future." *Burns & Trauma*, vol. 2, no. 4, Oct. 2014, pp. 169–80.
Lukács, Georg. *The Historical Novel*. 1937. Translated by Hannah Mitchell and Stanley Mitchell, Beacon, 1963.
MacLennan, Hugh. *Barometer Rising*. 1941. McClelland & Stewart, 1989.
Marais, Mike. "Violence, Postcolonial Fiction, and the Limits of Sympathy." *Studies in the Novel*, vol. 43, no. 1, 2011, pp. 94–114.
Mardorossian, Carine M. "What Is 'Worse Besides'? An Ecocritical Reading of Madness in Caribbean Literature." *Madness in Anglophone Caribbean Literature: On the Edge*, edited by Bénédicte Ledent et al., Springer, 2018, pp. 103–15.
McAllister, Margaret. "Nurse as Wounded Healer in *The English Patient*." *TEXT*, vol. 21, no. Special 38, Apr. 2017, pp. 1–14.
McDermott, Sinéad. "The Double Wound: Shame and Trauma in Joy Kogawa's *Obasan*." *Sexed Sentiments: Interdisciplinary Perspectives on Gender and Emotion*, edited by Willemijn Ruberg and Kristine Steenbergh, Rodopi, 2011, pp. 141–63.
McGonegal, Julie. *Imagining Justice: The Politics of Postcolonial Forgiveness and Reconciliation*. McGill-Queen's, 2009.
McVey, Christopher. "Reclaiming the Past: Michael Ondaatje and the Body of History." *Journal of Modern Literature*, vol. 37, no. 2, Winter 2014, pp. 141–60.

Metcalf, James. "*The English Patient*: Michael Ondaatje's Characterization of the Nurse-Patient Relationship." *Creative Nursing*, vol. 15, no. 1, 2009, pp. 28–30.
Minghella, Anthony, director. *The English Patient*. Miramax, 1996.
Montgomery, Adam. *Invisible Injured: Psychological Trauma in the Canadian Military from the First World War to Afghanistan*. McGill-Queen's, 2017.
Mootoo, Shani. *Cereus Blooms at Night*. Press Gang, 1996.
Mootoo, Shani. "On Becoming an Indian Starboy." *Canadian Literature*, no. 196, 2008, pp. 83–94.
Morrison, Toni. *Beloved*. Plume, 1987.
"Narrate, V." *Oxford English Dictionary*, Oxford UP, Mar. 2024.
Nestel, Sheryl. *Colour Coded Health Care the Impact of Race and Racism on Canadians' Health*. Wellesley Institute, 2012.
Nielsen, Emilia. "Transforming Disabling Trauma through Care Work and Collective Affinity: Mental Disability and 'a Shared Queerness' in *Cereus Blooms at Night*." *Studies in Canadian Literature*, vol. 44, no. 1, 2019, pp. 181–97.
O'Callaghan, Evelyn. "Sex, Secrets, and Shani Mootoo's Queer Families." *Contemporary Women's Writing*, vol. 6, no. 3, Nov. 2012, pp. 233–50.
Ondaatje, Michael. *The English Patient*. 1992. Vintage, 1993.
"Patient, adj. & n." *Oxford English Dictionary*, Oxford UP, Sept. 2024.
Pirbhai, Miriam. "Sexuality as (Counter) Discourse and Hybridity as Healing Practice in Shani Mootoo's *Cereus Blooms at Night*." *Journal of Caribbean Literatures*, vol. 4, no. 1, 2005, pp. 175–84.
Provencal, Vernon. "Sleeping with Herodotus in *The English Patient*." *Studies in Canadian Literature*, vol. 27, no. 2, 2002, pp. 140–59.
Ratliff, Ben. "They've Kidnapped 'The English Patient'." *The New York Times*, 23 Mar. 1997, p. 47.
Riemer, Heiko, and Rudolph Kuper. "Wadi Sura and the Gilf Kebir National Park-Challenge and Chance for Archaeology and Conservation in Egypt's Southwest." *Oasis Papers 6: Dakhleh Oasis Project Monograph 15*, edited by Roger S. Bagnall et al., Oxbow, 2012, pp. 107–17.
Robinson, Greg. *A Tragedy of Democracy: Japanese Confinement in North America*. Columbia UP, 2009.
Rose, Jonathan, editor. *The Holocaust and the Book: Destruction and Preservation*. U of Massachusetts P, 2001.
Rothberg, Michael. *Traumatic Realism: The Demands of Holocaust Representation*. U of Minnesota P, 2000.
Saeed, Humaira. "Postcolonial Sexualities and the Intelligibility of Dissidence." *The Bloomsbury Introduction to Postcolonial Writing*, edited by Jenni Ramone, Bloomsbury, 2017, pp. 237–54.
Scarry, Elaine. *The Body in Pain: The Making and Unmaking of the World*. Oxford UP, 1985.
Solecki, Sam. "Ondaatje, Michael." *The Oxford Companion to Canadian Literature*. 1997, Oxford UP, 2006.
Sontag, Susan. *Regarding the Pain of Others*. Picador, 2003.
Visvis, Vikki. "Traumatic Representation: The Power and Limitations of Storytelling as 'Talking Cure' in Michael Ondaatje's *In the Skin of a Lion* and *The English Patient*." *Ariel*, vol. 40, no. 4, 2009, pp. 89–108.
Webb, Peter. "'At War with Nature': Animals in Timothy Findley's *The Wars*." *Other Selves Animals in the Canadian Literary Imagination*, edited by Janice Anne Fiamengo, U of Ottawa P, 2007, pp. 227–44.
Wells-Lassagne, Shannon, and Fiona McMahon, editors. *Adapting Margaret Atwood*. Springer, 2021.

Williams, David. "A Force of Interruption: The Photography of History in Timothy Findley's *The Wars*." *Canadian Literature*, no. 194, Autumn 2007, pp. 54–73.
Winterson, Jeanette. *Written on the Body*. Jonathan Cape, 1992.
York, Lorraine. *The Other Side of Dailiness: Photography in the Works of Alice Munro, Timothy Findley, Michael Ondaatje, and Margaret Laurence*. ECW, 1988.

3

MENTAL AFFLICTION, AUTOBIOGRAPHY, AND THE LITERARY HISTORY OF ASSISTED DEATH

Mental affliction forms perhaps the most recurrent medical theme in Canadian literature. This chapter takes a broad view of ailments of the brain, ranging from disability to depictions of mental illness and addiction among non-Indigenous Canadians, to consider how literature about disorders of the mind illuminates the limits of language, autobiographical impulses, and the literary history of medical assistance in dying (MAID) in Canada.

I begin with a discussion of how authors' biographies have combatted stigma around mental illness and how a conjunction between the poets Earle Birney and Al Purdy establishes a literary background for provisions of MAID. I next move to a reading of *Boy in the Moon* (2009), Ian Brown's memoir of caring for a child with an impossibly rare syndrome, before discussing addiction in Jowita Bydlowska's memoir, *Drunk Mom* (2013), and Vincent Lam's *On the Ravine* (2023), and closing with Miriam Toews's account of a family impacted by depression and suicide in *All My Puny Sorrows* (2014). While MAID is currently not provided to people suffering from mental illness, literature about the mind illuminates the cultural history of this procedure in Canada.

The works addressed in this chapter are all either autobiographical or close to it, with Lam's novel built from his experiences as an addiction physician, and they were all published within the last fifteen years. As a result, in addition to their exploration of key themes of mental ailment and illness, these books also reflect a rising cultural interest in nonfiction narrative and offer deeply personal accounts of afflictions that often defy communication. As Neil Vickers outlines, autobiographical accounts of illness have drawn the attention of many critics and theorists, including

DOI: 10.4324/9781003340119-4

Einat Avrahami, Thomas Couser, Arthur W. Frank, and Anne Hunsaker Hawkins. Hawkins argues that memoirs of sickness can be understood as their own category of writing, which she calls "pathography." The works included in this chapter invite readers to question autobiographical motives in writing about the mind.

Other works that treat the mind beyond the focus of this chapter include those concerning later-life dementia, which has been such a frequent theme in Canadian literature that a monograph by Marlene Goldman focuses solely on the topic. Goldman traces the Canadian cultural history of Alzheimer's and age-related cognitive impairment through their Gothic and apocalyptic portrayals in literature. Celebrated Canadian works in this category include Margaret Laurence's *The Stone Angel* (1964), Mordecai Richler's *Barney's Version* (1997), and Alice Munro's story "The Bear Came Over the Mountain" (2001). All three have been made into motion pictures, demonstrating their perceived cultural significance. The mystery writer Howard Engel's memoir, *The Man Who Forgot How to Read* (2007), offers an interesting portrayal of a literary mind recuperating from stroke, while Rohinton Mistry depicts an elderly character with Parkinson's disease in *Family Matters* (2002). The filmmaker Sarah Polley's book of essays *Run Towards the Danger* (2022) includes a noteworthy account of her recovery from concussion. Readers looking for writing on such neurological conditions should seek out these works.

Alistair MacLeod's *No Great Mischief* (1999) doesn't centre addiction to the same extent as the works discussed at more length here, but it also represents an important Canadian portrayal of alcoholism. A bestseller, the novel won the Dublin IMPAC prize, a major international award (Fuller). *No Great Mischief* repeatedly focalizes the cultural significance of and at times overreliance on whisky among the Scottish Canadian men whose lives it portrays. Cheryl Lousley points out that responses to MacLeod's work tend to focus on the beauty of his depiction "of labouring men who honour their craft, their place, and their kin, even as that honourable world disappears" (239). A key activity of these men in this work of honouring and mourning is drinking whisky. The novel can be read as a chronicle of alcoholism and should be remembered when surveying representations of addiction in Canadian literature.

Mental Illness and Addiction, Medical Assistance in Dying (MAID), and Literary History

In reading literature about the mind, it's important to consider how many Canadian authors have lived with mental illness and addiction, and how many have died by suicide or accessed assisted death. Authors have both drawn creative capacity from their neurodiversity, and had their personal experiences publicized to combat stigma. In a literary biography that also documents a late-twentieth-century history of addiction treatment in Toronto, Rosemary Sullivan recounts the influential poet Gwendolyn MacEwen's many hospitalizations and early death due to alcohol addiction at age forty-seven. In 2010, Robert Munsch, the author of nearly one hundred children's books that have sold an astounding eighty-two million copies (Scholastic), disclosed his decades-long work to live with addiction and mental illness (Munsch, and Row). Irene Gammel points out that Lucy Maud Montgomery is thought to have composed *Anne of Green Gables* at a time of elevated mood (85), which alternated with the severe lows that ultimately claimed her life: in 2008, her granddaughter revealed Montgomery's intentional fatal overdose at age sixty-seven (Gammel 84). Disclosing suicide as the cause of death combats stigma, thereby making it easier for others suffering from mental illness to access life-saving help. These examples reflect the thoughtful leveraging of literary fame to support an important cause and show that many Canadian authors have suffered with mental illness and addiction. The stories of their personal lives can offer sources of hope and inspiration.

While the publication of these authors' biographies combats stigma, literary history also gives a backdrop to Canada's 2016 legalization of medical assistance in dying (MAID). Two major court cases in the 1990s impacted Canadian impressions of assisted death and offer important context for interpreting this cultural development: Sue Rodriguez's failed 1993 request that the Supreme Court grant her an assisted death to end her suffering from amyotrophic lateral sclerosis (ALS), and Robert Latimer's 1994 and 1997 trials for the murder of his twelve-year-old daughter, Tracy, who lived with severe and painful disabilities (see Duffin 468–71), a story referenced in Ian Brown's book.

A convergence between two poets, Earle Birney and Al Purdy, illustrates a literary background to these 1990s conversations that contributed to the legalization of MAID. Birney's narrative poem "David" (1942) recounts the assisted death of a hiker and was included in his Governor General's Award-winning collection by the same title. Frequently reprinted in anthologies and read in schools, the work's themes of mercy and tragedy may be among the most memorialized of any Canadian poem after "In Flanders Fields." Two young friends climb a mountain in the poem, but when David falls after losing his footing and is paralyzed, he begs and finally persuades Bob to push him over a ledge to end his life, saying "I'd do it for you, Bob" (152). Birney bookends this incident with the killing and deaths of animals. In two foreshadowing discoveries, the friends come upon a skeleton on a rock that teaches Bob "that a goat could slip" (44) and later they find a robin with a broken wing, which David kills, asking, "Could you teach it to fly?" (64). As Bob tears down the mountain after David's death, he says, "My feet squelched a slug and horror/Rose again in my nostrils" (177–78). The destruction of a much humbler creature offers a conduit to Bob's emotions about his act. Reminiscent of Samuel Taylor Coleridge's "The Rime of the Ancient Mariner" (1834), Birney's long poem explores themes of guilt, compassion, and culpability through a parallel focus on what humans owe to animals, creatures that people use to imagine the limits of humanity, in order to question whether killing out of mercy is inhuman or humane.

In 1974, the major Canadian poet Al Purdy, a younger friend of Birney's, published a commentary on the themes of assisted death in "David" ("The Man Who Killed David") that offers context to his own later decision to access medical assistance in dying. Showing the enduring presence of the poem in the younger poet's consciousness, twenty years after publishing this article, in a 1996 essay on his late friend, Purdy described his production of a CBC radio adaptation of "David," writing that "the ghosts who inhabit that poem still float through my head" ("Earle Birney"). The next year Purdy joined the Right to Die Society founded by activist John Hofsess, and, in 2000, suffering from a variety of ailments at age 81, he accessed an assisted death with the activist's help (Hofsess). The service was still illegal at that time and risked prosecution for murder. In a 2016 essay timed to appear just after his own assisted death, Hofsess revealed the poet's choice with his prior blessing a few months before MAID was officially legalized in Canada, arguing that the stigma around mental illness and suicide slowed public acceptance of the procedure.

Reactions to this announcement echoed the media attention given the 1997 news that the author Margaret Laurence had also opted for an assisted death ten years earlier (Smith). The conjunction between these authors' stories and the history of MAID reveals how one thread of a national conversation on "mercy killing" that changed both Canadian law and public consciousness travelled through literature. It also illustrates how authors can use their status, as public figures, to advance ethical agendas with national impacts.

From the national soul-searching occasioned by the 1990s Rodriguez and Latimer trials and the lasting celebration of Birney's poem to Purdy's covert assisted death and the legalization of MAID, Canadian concepts of merciful death have developed in tandem with literary history. Part of what's at stake in these cultural narratives is how assisted dying looks different depending on the ailment and state of the patient. Capacity to consent is now an enshrined requirement for MAID that was not as evident during Latimer's prosecution. Still, thorny complexities remain in official guidance to physicians in determining whether a desire for MAID is suicidal ideation (see CAMH and Health Canada), and when and whether acquiescing to such desires is or is not ethical.

Published two years before the legalization of MAID, Toews's *All My Puny Sorrows* struggles with whether seemingly incurable depression warrants assisted death, a question touched on in Amy Rushton's discussion of the novel. In her nuanced reading of this idea in the book, Sabrina Reed explains that "Toews takes on not only her own reluctance to condone the death of a much-loved sister but also the Canadian justice system's infantilization of the mentally ill" (188). With the government of Canada postponing access to MAID based on mental illness until 2027 to allow for further expert consideration (Kirkup), patients with what they view as terminal depression are seeking court injunctions to give them access to this procedure, sometimes in disputes with their families (Tait and Anderssen), with other avenues risking lasting pain and even prosecution. As this chapter explores through stories about ailments of the mind at various stages of life, the lessons of literature illuminate without always resolving such moral thickets.

Disability: Ian Brown's *Boy in the Moon* (2009)

The Boy in the Moon (2009) is the journalist Ian Brown's account of learning how to look after his son, Walker, who was born with cardiofaciocutaneous (CFC) syndrome and who lives with severe mental and physical disabilities as a result. Brown's story is a quest to understand the limits of Walker's access to dignity and selfhood in the eyes of a world that must also learn to care for him. Ailments of the mind raise questions regarding what makes illness, whether it must be contagious, or is indicated simply in the presence of pain, or whether illness inheres in some impossible-to-define "abnormality." Walker's chronic pain alone might seem to make him ill, but Brown implicitly questions whether you can be ill if you are living with a condition with which you were born and for which there is no cure.

Though not a work of fiction, Brown's realist depiction of the details of caring for his son is profoundly literary, as its excavation of character uses language to strive to transcend language. Brown's text was partly generated through serialization of his newspaper columns (292), which allows his prose to log a level of detail rarely achieved in retrospective memoirs. From the built-up crust of spilled formula on his carpet (2), to his acute familiarity with the benefits of stacking bins (21), the result is an accumulation of detail that chronicles the desperation and banality of caring for a profoundly uncommon child. His ongoing work as a journalist for *The Globe and Mail* has let Brown periodically extend the story of *Boy in the Moon* with updates on his life with Walker, for example in an essay on the perseverance of their relationship through the social distancing of the COVID-19 pandemic ("Two Metres"). As Amelia DeFalco points out, Brown's book captures his "longing to apprehend his son's subjectivity" (37) and can be read according to Thomas Couser's notion of "somatography," writing that contends with another person's life in an unusual body (29). Widely discussed and celebrated abroad and at home (DeFalco 36), Brown's book should be considered within the canon of Canadian prose narrative.

An important context for this book is the innovation of the L'Arche communities for people with mental disabilities. Founded by Canadian Jean Vanier, scion of an influential political family whose father served as the first French-Canadian governor general (Monet), the system of international homes creates community for people with disabilities where they may live on their own terms. Brown struggles with his family's ultimate decision to place their son in care, but the example of L'Arche seems to offer a way forward. Jean Vanier was later revealed to have sexually abused dozens of residents at the homes he founded, a tragedy that Brown covered for *The Globe and Mail* ("L'Arche"). Brown's work should also be understood in historical relation to the national conversations about the rights and dignity of people living with disabilities sparked by the death of Tracy Latimer. Commenting on the case and the desperation of caregivers without social support, another parent of a child with CFC tells Brown, "we're all complicit in Tracy's death" (270). At birth, when Walker doesn't start breathing on his own and only major interventions keep him alive, Brown wonders "Had the doctor been asking me if I wanted to let Walker's life end, as nature would have ended it on its own?" (26). This prospect of a death that doctors permit by doing nothing should be read in the context of assisted death. Medical professionals can stop procedures at the end of life because patients can consent to the withholding of care. But infants, for whom there are massive interventions available, yet who may go on to live in agony in worlds that do not accommodate their difference, have only their parents as advocates, people operating with incomplete knowledge. Brown charts the weight of this relation.

His book traces two overarching challenges: first is Walker's effort to thrive given his profound deficits. The second is Brown's work to come to terms with the significance of his child's birth and the meaning of his life, the question of what kind of mind belongs to his son. Brown, an author, is forced to confront the failures of language itself in the mouths of doctors, of friends and family struggling to empathize, and in his own voice as he faces his desperation to connect with his son. Throughout the text, Brown questions how best to understand Walker's needs, and seeks out a variety of social frameworks for accommodating unusual children, from disability rights advocates who might insist on integration, to doctors who, in their race to save an infant's life, turn a blind eye to the desperation survival itself can engender. Brown explores the brutality of forcing people not able to fully participate in society to live in relation to social norms. He emphasizes at every turn what his son teaches him about the power of being confronted by limits, about learning to live in the moment, and discovering new ways to value being alive.

Brown's book superimposes his effort to find meaning in life on his effort to understand Walker and his syndrome that has placed him in a world of pain. Brown writes that "What I cared about was whether he had a sense of himself, an inner life. Sometimes it seemed like the most urgent question of all" (48). Yet Walker's life is excruciating, and the question of his inner world is superseded by the evidence of his constant pain. His father is perpetually distracted by his cries, "the sound of his steady agony" (49), and describes him as "A boxer, a tough guy," who "may be tiny, but he is rugged, and has a bottomless capacity for pain" (239). Walker's likes "feel like accomplishments" (241) and when he "does anything to suggest there's a point to his life besides pain and isolation, it seems particularly brave" (242). Johanna, Walker's mother, struggles with this state of his life, the question of his life's value, and the problem his continuous suffering poses to finding an answer (182–83). Brown too ruminates over these questions, writing that "I was always looking for a context in which to make sense of Walker, in which his disorganized life (and my unavoidable devotion to it) might take on more meaning and purpose" (157). The book is Brown's excavation and creation of context, his note-taking as he sets about trying to gain perspective on his son, whether his affliction is illness, a wrongness in his body, or whether it is Brown himself who is not at first equipped to see him as sufficient.

For Brown, this disorganized life caused by Walker's disability is in fact clarifying. He writes, "Walker is a lens—one with an unusual shape, I admit—through which to see the world more sharply" (242). This lens, Brown says, gives him "a longer view" (167). Reflecting on Charles de Gaulle's devotion to his own disabled child, Brown sees "the gaunt, spare shape of our human loneliness and longing clarified by his simplified child" (233). For Brown, children with disabilities sharpen the perspectives of their caregivers. Brown comes to find that accepting the meaning of his son's life as it is helps him see the meaning of his own existence, writing that "Walker was himself; he had no choice. If I could let him be the boy he was, and let go of the boy he might have been—maybe I could do the same" (194). Despite Walker's immense troubles and the burden of caring for him, Brown finds in parenting this child the relief of "a destiny I couldn't avoid" (27), and says, "Life with him and life without him: both were unthinkable" (68). Brown does ultimately find meaning in Walker's life and writes that the boy

> is proof of what the imperfect and the fragile have to offer; a reminder that there are many ways to be human; a concentrator of joy; an insistent nudge to pay attention to every passing mote of daily life that otherwise slips by uncounted.
>
> *(180)*

Brown does find meaning in Walker's life through the child's push to intensify attention.

This push is wordless, and Brown, a writer, focuses on the stakes of this communication beyond language, while words fail again and again. Walker cannot speak, but "Tone, inflection, implication: he got all that. He was a master of the unspoken" (252). The father and son find their own way to communicate. "As he grew older," Brown writes, "we developed a private language of tongue clicks that only he and I speak" (34). Clicks offer a shared vocabulary, and, as Brown writes, "Walker and I don't compound our confusion with words. We prefer noises" (246). Sometimes his parents find meaning in even the repetitive pain of watching Walker hit himself: "At other times he seemed to do it more expressively, as a way to clear his head, or to let us know he would be saying something if he could talk" (77). The lack of communication impacts the parents of disabled children, who can be easily spotted at Walker's daycare because "They were starved for contact and longing to tell the truth" (47). Part of the challenge of communicating with Walker comes from the disconnect between his experience of the world and his parents'. Brown explores a painting analogy to explain his effort to see order and detail in his son that is not part of the blank canvas of his world (42). His parents struggle to accept that their desire for communicable details in Walker's world does not reflect its reality. During a visit to Disney World, a land of themes, Brown writes, "Walker keeps reminding me that life does not have a theme" (236):

> His screaming had been non-stop for an hour, and under the relentless steamy Florida sun had expanded in my head to the point where the human agony it represented, the displacement and existential isolation it represented, were the only things I could hear or think about or even see.
>
> *(238)*

For the author, trained in leveraging the full spectrum of language for his goals, the most brutal recognition is that his son's only way to relay the meaning of his life—both for practical and, it seems, expressive reasons—is through a single nonverbal utterance, a scream.

Throughout Brown's book, the question of whether congenital disability is illness hovers, whether Walker is abnormal and suffering from a problem whose cure or solution is theoretically clear, or whether he is simply himself, an impossibly rare version of being human. Brown points out that his society's resistance to assimilating Walker's version of normal may reveal its own deformity. As a mother of daughters with disabilities reflects,

> I look at the girls, and I think, Who's to say they're not happier in their world than I am in mine? And here I am feeling sorry for them because I'm trying to judge them by the standards of the world they aren't part of.
>
> (144)

Brown uses the contrived landscape of a theme park to frame this insight in his own terms, saying that he imagines in Disney World he feels "the way Walker feels in the real world: it has its charms, but mostly we don't quite fit" (237). This sense of the failure of society to accommodate difference defines the author's contemplation of housing options for his son. In Brown's view, the history of efforts to care for people with mental disabilities reveals a broad social "discomfort with the irrational, or struggle with what frightens us, our longing to control what we encounter" (263). Finding a new living situation for Walker means finding a social landscape that normalizes his reality. Brown contends with the challenges in discovering, creating, and maintaining a place for his son that could be at once a professionally managed facility and a home (186). When he is placed "In his new vacation home, as I think of it," Brown writes, "surrounded by peers, he's as solid as anyone. I hope that is the gift we gave him by giving him up" (109). Finding him a home means finding him a social reality where he is understood to be not ill, but normal.

The social stakes of this work of normalizing relationships is a primary theme of the book. Brown writes of meeting a child with the same syndrome as Walker who "often approaches strangers on the street. 'Hi,' he says. 'Do you like me?' That's the real question" (126). When he started working with people with disabilities, Vanier, too, found they all seemed to ask, "Do you love me? And, will you be my friend?" (203). Brown repeats and restates these questions posed by people with disabilities (284), as they underpin how social worlds respond to their presence. People living at L'Arche, Brown writes, "didn't seem to suffer from the self-consciousness the rest of us do: disabled or not, they launched forthwith into the act of 'relationship' with whomever they met, whenever they met them" (197). This act of relationship is constant for everyone striving to live within a society, but Brown points out how the lack of accommodation of people with disabilities forces them to keep posing the question, to demand a response. Through this ethical work to relate, Brown finds profound social lessons. "Every ounce of me knows my odd little boy can teach everyone something about themselves," Brown concludes, but "Whether that will ever happen is another story" (211). This act of relation is educating, and the lessons people with disabilities have to teach in this domain are profound, but frequently ignored.

Brown investigates the limits of scientific knowledge and the value of diagnosis as a form of insight. Walker is diagnosed as having cardiofaciocutaneous (CFC) syndrome in his first year of life (30–31), but when genetic testing for the disorder becomes available, he doesn't have the DNA markers (171). His family finds an explanation and community in the circle of parents of children who at last looked just like Walker (112–57), and yet the biological checkmark is withheld. The author's search to better understand his son's mind culminates in the devastation of a long sought-after and long-delayed MRI (275–76), when he finally sees an anatomical explanation for what his son lacks: multiple components of Walker's brain are far smaller than they should be (278–79). The sight both explains everything and is another mystery, as the neurologist lacks words to fully explain the MRI results (277). Despite the brilliance of the children's hospital, a site he knows "like I knew my own basement" (63), "the place was filled with doctors who couldn't help my boy" (63). While he says of a scientist that "optimism is the default position of his profession" (282), Brown's own skepticism

> tended to show itself after the fourth doctor in a row told me something I already knew. Sometimes they saw my skepticism and agreed with it, quietly admitting their own helplessness, which made me like them again. Sometimes they spotted my frustration, and stayed away.
>
> *(63)*

The best doctors admit the limits of their knowledge, while optimism and skepticism represent orientations towards the unknown that can divide patients and families from scientists. Optimism implies a position of hope, whereas scepticism suggests a position of negative expectation. Brown relates most easily to physicians who remain open to their patients' scepticism, while ideally maintaining their own optimism.

Throughout the book, Brown contends with the extent and limits of knowledge promised by genetic science. Touching on the idea that genetic analysis dehumanizes people by dispelling the mystery of the body (273), Brown suggests that "In a genetics lab, Walker would always be a deleterious effect of nature and evolution, and little more" (177). He writes that "Genetic tests are a way to eliminate the imperfect, all the pain and agony that comes with that imperfection" (80). Though he once "spent part of every day furiously wishing that a test had been available, wishing that we had had a choice in the matter of his existence, for his sake and our own as well" (180), he comes to question "if the prospect of looking after a disabled child did not threaten to destroy the lives of those doing the caring—if we had such alternatives, would we need a test at all?" (180) While Brown contends with the meaning and value of genetic testing in advance of birth, the detail and clarity of genetic science reveals a further horizon of unknowing. Acknowledging the role of technology in his survival and endurance, Brown observes that Walker is not "a product of nature alone" (167), yet, Brown points out that "the technology was more advanced than any scientific understanding of what the technology revealed" (169). In a footnote, he asks, "Does an oversimplified model of how a human being comes to be result in an oversimplified model of what a human being is?" (178). With so little understood about the real workings of the genome, Brown reveals the search for definitive answers to be as futile as expecting Walker to start talking instead of relating to others on his own terms.

Brown's shifting orientations toward the unknown point to one of his main topics—the question of the extent to which Walker himself can be known. "Without a knowable brain," Brown asks, "was Walker a knowable boy? If he wasn't knowable, what was his value?" (282). Social expectations regarding the value of a life often presume that others must understand it. Brown's book has been critiqued for reissuing notions of cognitive ability as a measure of human value (DeFalco 38), but, as DeFalco argues, its conclusion shows that Walker's "unassimilable difference is no longer a source of distress for Brown" (41), who finds a way to express how his son's value and difference both exceed explanation (42). Brown's circling questions regarding his son's knowability correspond to the broad issue of how narrative can and cannot bring greater knowledge.

Though he struggles towards answers to the questions of whether Walker's affliction could be alleviated if not cured, the story itself reveals the illness in how the rest of the world fails to accommodate him. The state of not knowing, Brown realizes, is not unique to parenting a child with disabilities, since he writes, "the average father doesn't know a lot of the time if he and his sons aren't making up their bond either" (246). Even as scientists try and fail to contextualize Walker, for Brown, the boy himself offers clarification and his own kind of insight: "He is the antidote to false consciousness. He will always remind me of where we truly are" (238). Brown's conclusion offers a simple insight, the most important knowledge in a field of unknowing about his son: "I knew I loved him, and I knew he knew it" (288). Knowledge of loving and being loved, the answer to the question all people with disabilities seem to ask in this book, is the most important awareness of all.

Addiction: Jowita Bydlowska's *Drunk Mom* (2013) and Vincent Lam's *On the Ravine* (2023)

Two works from the last decade help frame notions of addiction in Canadian prose narrative. Whereas Vincent Lam's *On the Ravine* (2023) offers an unprecedented medical perspective on opioid dependency, Jowita Bydlowska's *Drunk Mom* (2013) presents a rare view of how addiction impacts motherhood.

Published the same year as Canadian journalist Ann Dowsett Johnston's bestselling *Drink: The Intimate Relationship Between Women and Alcohol* (2013), Bydlowska's memoir uncovers a gendered experience of alcohol dependency. As Dagmara Drewniak points out, Bydlowska's work of memoir and life writing combines efforts to write about both addiction and motherhood at once. *Drunk Mom* explores wanting as a feeling akin to a mother's desire for her baby, and the infant's need of a parent. "This is the wanting that has no end" (40), she writes. "It's a baby—a wet, hungry baby that no one is picking up to soothe" (4). She brings the analogy from her craving to her own self: "I'm exactly like a baby" (5). So immense are her cravings that she pursues them even as she plans to seek help: "To prepare for rehab, I watch the TV show about addiction, *Intervention*. I watch it night after night, on my computer—while I drink" (154). As she ridicules the name of Toronto's Centre for Addiction and Mental Health (48), gets rid of empties along with formula (74), reads dependency memoirs and a textbook about addictions (77–78), she wonders if her doctor ever had a drug addiction, maybe in medical school (104), like Vincent Lam's Fitz. "Alcoholism is not drinking, just like hemophilia is not bleeding" (14), she writes, while a counsellor argues against relying on labels and identities such as "alcoholic," instead of seeking to understand tendencies (60).

Bydlowska uses the permanence of limbs to describe her dependency, writing that "My addiction is also a body part. I can't get rid of it any easier than I can cut off my own arm or poke my eye out" (99). Likewise, when she manages to sleep without drinking first, "It is like wrapping an amputation in bandages, but at least I've stopped the bleeding" (101). Circumventing free will, the addiction feels as internal as lungs: "There are no decisions; the action will be prompted by an involuntary muscle, a breath going in and out" (113). She suggests that "it's not the addiction that I try to figure out but the thing that makes people addicts" (154), coming to believe that what they all share is that "We'll always understand what it's like to be afraid to wake up" (286). Reflecting on time and addiction, how cravings alter experiences of duration, she writes that "In a way, my seven months is less than five days" (285). The book chronicles group therapy and the trauma patients discuss (187–90), as well as injuries Bydlowska suffers through the course of her addiction (247–50). Bydlowska treats the question of cure with delicacy: "I believe you're never cured of alcoholism. I use the word *cure* because it is not strictly a disease . . . Disease implies you can maybe cure it" (14). Late in the book when she goes to a meeting, as a sign of healing, she writes that "The wanting is as strong as always. But now it's for the right thing" (253).

The intractability of substance dependency and the shifting hope for healing, if not a cure, also define addictions physician Vincent Lam's novel *On the Ravine* (2023). The book dramatizes the dilemmas of the opioid crisis, an ongoing tragedy that doesn't always make the news (3)—or literature. The title is a parable for the brink of addiction and refers to the "crumbling house on the edge of the ravine" (266) where Fitz, a former doctor, gives fixes to users. Increasingly dilapidated since Fitz lost his license because of his own addiction, the house is in Toronto's wealthy Rosedale neighbourhood, which borders an extensive valley wilderness. Lam's novelistic argument for a safe supply explores what happens between doctors and patients, those trying often at once to help or be helped. Both often find themselves at the precipice of the deeper, darker "downs" of being high, while the messiness of distinctions between doctors and patients, medications and street drugs, the desire to empathize and the need for boundaries, represent the many slippery slopes Lam's characters face on the ravine.

Lam's textured chronicle of the life of an addictions doctor is Dickensian in its focus on urban social fabric and the sometimes-noxious idiosyncrasies of characters, as when Chen must maintain professionalism towards a racist patient (168–74). Lam also details illnesses of withdrawal, the practicalities and intricacies of drug use and addictions treatment, and the risks of homelessness and petty crime that result from addiction. The novel scrutinizes the lessons in humility and complexity that doctors need, the role of the doctor–patient relationship in bringing about both cures and care, and the logic of addiction, which often makes people sick whether or not they can access the drugs they crave. Throughout Lam compares the grey ethics of both legal and illicit drug industries, and the simultaneous inevitability and futility of attempts at altruism. The book opens with Chen looking through a folder of photos he keeps of dead patients (1–3). As he writes to his former student, "Within the picture of addiction, I told you, figures are hidden in the shadows" (41). The book represents an attempt to pull these faces out of the shadows, to cast light on one figure in particular, Claire, while also revealing the struggles of those trying to care for her.

Lam's novel regards Toronto through the opioid crisis and attends to differences between neighbourhoods like Kensington Market and Rosedale, even as Chen often bikes through the city visiting suffering people throughout the ravines (8–12). The book could be read as a map of Toronto through the opioid crisis, contrasting the spaces of the clinic, drug house, and hospital. Chen arrives at Fitz's house through the ravine (12), a space given over to wilderness within the city's infrastructure that occupies a kind of netherworld within Toronto's consciousness of itself. Whereas Chen has set up an addictions clinic in Kensington Market (14), after leaving medicine due to his alcoholism (21), Fitz has let his house in the expensive neighbourhood of Rosedale become a kind of grassroots safe injection site, where people can use substances under his medically trained watch and dying is not allowed (17). This permissive space is in fact safer than use in the streets. Lam's clinical expertise allows him to explore the tension between allowing users to dose with a safe supply versus withholding their preferred drugs as they finish treatment (18). Whereas Lam's other work has foregrounded the space of the hospital, this novel contrasts Fitz's house with Chen's clinic as portals for caring for people who are otherwise filtering on their own through the city facing greater and greater risks.

Like a medical history, Lam's narrative of Claire's addiction charts the arrival of the problem and her effort to escape. He explains her early dependence on opioids for pain relief after an injury (60), and her introduction to heroin as a stronger high (65). Chen asks her whether there was "anything else they helped you with, in addition to the pain" (68), since dependencies may stem from emotional as well as physical cravings. For Claire, music is the "most important thing" (68), and Chen tries to persuade her that beating the addiction could enhance rather than steal her unique musicality: "*You play so well despite the pain, despite the drugs. Imagine if we can help you*, he wanted to say, *the music you would make*" (52). Despite her treatment she starts using again in advance of a performance (185). Chen attends and is awestruck by her talent but knows she's relapsed: "In clinic, he would have told his patient, 'You could play like this without using whatever you took,' wanting to believe it, and to persuade his patient to believe it as well" (188). But at the concert, faced with the splendour of her intoxicated playing, he can't believe sobriety would let her play as well, and he discusses the ethics of his quandary with Fitz (189). Chen's student also loved Claire's playing at the restaurant they always went to together (188, 267), and he realized she was also a user when she returned from the bathroom one night free of the cold symptoms he hadn't realized were the result of withdrawal (212). His student "had once told Chen that she wished she could exist within a moment of beauty as Claire did—that that would be enough for her" (267). These characters with addictions are connected through their dangerous desire for a transcendent oblivion. At the end of the novel, when Chen finds Claire again after hearing a violin, she says she's no longer using (356). The fact that her music now is "sweet, brightly coloured, but with nothing hidden or uniquely expressive" (354) seems like proof of her sobriety. Later he hears wild playing again through the city blocks, Claire's music as he remembers it, but it's only a recording (357). Like an analogy for the limits and openings of empathy itself, Lam uses sound to give Chen a conduit to Claire's world, both emotionally and in the streets, a space he can be aware of but not always access. Hearing music through the city offers Lam a way to dramatize the lost-and-found connection between Chen and his patient, as well as evidence of the losses she endures through the course of her addiction and treatment.

Lam traces the question of how doctors proffering medication do or do not differ from dealers, and where drug companies fit in this scheme. "Just like a good dealer," Claire thinks of Chen as he offers her treatment for her addiction, "he's pushing me to have a little more" (85), though she eventually no longer thinks of Chen as a dealer (178). Lam also depicts Claire's relations with the pharmacists managing her treatment (87–88), in another reflection of official providers taking on the role of dealer. Fitz is known as the "dealing doctor" (241), but he prefers "wholesaler" in providing the safe supply he offers (17). Chen is acutely aware of moments when his prescriptions killed (4), and, as he watches a drug deal, he wonders "Who was buying and who was selling" (5), which remains a constant question throughout the book. Amid these muddy distinctions between dealers and doctors, Lam places the corporate motivations of the drug trial. The company pushing it, Varitas, may be seeking cures for addiction, but is also mixing greed with the desire to bring new consumables to patients, and in that sense represents another dealer looking to exploit their suffering. In his affair with the drug company representative, Bella, Chen doesn't know "whether she's using me, or I'm using her" (189). Lam scrutinizes the stakes of using and being used for doctors, patients, and those with vested interests in their lives, whether dealers, drug reps, or enablers.

The agent who most enables Claire's addiction is her sister, Molly. The name "Molly" is a slang term for Ecstasy or MDMA, a common party drug that is sometimes seen as a gateway to more intense substances, though the evidence is mixed (Reid et al.). This trait reflects the impact of Molly as a character, which is to bring Claire further and further into a path of addiction through an avenue that at first just seems like fun. As children the sisters pursued advanced musical education, and traded accolades for time with their parents (149). Molly comes to visit Claire and seems disappointed that she's getting sober, as it was partly through her influence that Claire started using (155–58). Claire takes heroin again after finding Molly is using at their apartment, and, as a result, it seems, a musical collaborator likes her playing (182). To secure money for drugs, Claire and Molly turn to shoplifting (194–95), but having been paid in drugs, Claire needs to use naloxone on Molly to revive her (201). Chen persuades Fitz not to give Molly any more fentanyl patches to protect Claire (236), but as a result Molly accesses a large stash of heroin, which she and Claire start dealing (241). Lam thus tracks Chen's struggle to help his patient, and the greater benefit Fitz is sometimes able to achieve through the moral grey area of his own supplying operations.

Lam's text offers a detailed portrait of the ethical quandaries practitioners face in hunting for cures alongside large drug companies. Much of the book is given over to Chen's participation in the trial of a fictional drug called memorex. He meets at length with company executives (75–77), and has an affair with one (145). The drug itself has similar properties to psychedelic mushrooms (95) but has another biological source—lizards (99, 104). This substance may represent a stand-in for ayahuasca, a psychoactive South American mixture that has gained mainstream popularity in recent years. Its medicinal properties are replicated in Lam's ayahuagaine, of which memorex is the brand name for a presumptively pure and clean version (104). Though his addictions have blown his own involvement in the trial (96–97), Fitz has a talent for the recruitment of subjects (99) and helps Chen find users for the memorex trial (231). This process culminates in Claire's participation, which Chen ultimately tries but fails to stop: being a trial doctor above all (321–22) obliges him to prioritize large numbers over individual cases. Though her heart stops during the experiment (323), she had looked up traditional uses of the drug, so she "concentrated really hard on what I wanted to find, my truth. And now something is different. I feel free, and true" (324). Yet she still seems to need opiates for playing. She practises for hours (329), "But her favourite pieces lacked something" (332)—something essential had gone from her playing, "And she missed it" (332). Chen feels the need to report the "serious adverse event" of Claire's heart stopping (325) but goes against the will of his big pharma collaborators in doing so (328). When they use a technicality to negate the adverse finding (335), they persuade Chen to sign a nondisclosure agreement in exchange for a sum he doesn't feel he can refuse (339).

Again and again, Lam calls Chen's professionalism into question, as he checks on Claire when not technically permitted, in reporting the problem, and then in agreeing to be muzzled, reflecting how even good doctors are also bad. Molly and Claire enrol in the new study, but Molly breaks the rules by getting high right before their dosage (344–45). Whereas Claire is given a placebo (350) and seems to benefit from the presence of Chen as her trusted caregiver in administering the treatment, Molly receives the full medication and stops breathing as a result (347). The company rep Bella, Chen's occasional lover, flees the scene of Molly's death (350) to visit and, it seems, "use" Chen (350). Claire feels she's responsible for Molly's death (355) but Chen knows that "Whatever had happened, it was not her fault" (355): he could have stopped it by refusing to sell his silence. The drug trial permits the search for a promising cure for addiction, but the ethics lack clarity, and the costs may be too high.

While this book chronicles addictions, it is especially a story about Chen's orientation to the profession, and sense of himself as a doctor faced with impossible decisions. In explaining his reason for refusing to write a reference letter for a patient at the outset of the book, he says, "It's about my integrity" (3), offering one way of summarizing the novel itself. His relationship with the medical student with addiction to whom he writes throughout the book coalesces these struggles (6–7, 115, 164–67). In an echo of Fitz's story, this medical worker Chen admires turns out to have needed treatment as much as anyone else in his practice. His first discovery of the student's addiction seems like an "accounting problem" (239) that "involved a large quantity of missing opioids" (239). Chen also uses Fitz as a compass for his professionalism. While Fitz calls Chen for antibiotics (261), they argue over the fentanyl patches Fitz supplies (225), calling into question which one of them is "over the line" (226). Fitz thinks he's saving lives by "providing what they need," but Chen wants data (228), showing the problem of offering a safe supply without regulation and study. Despite his stance of disapproval toward his tactics, Chen uses Fitz as a moral compass, while his own behaviour tends to cross boundaries in relation to Claire. When Claire will be evicted (216–27), Chen offers to pay her rent (218), and then lets her stay in his condo (275). His difficulty in maintaining professional limits in relation to her shows one way of interpreting why this patient in particular is the main character of this story. When Chen brings Claire to Fitz when he realizes she's been selling contaminated drugs that have caused overdoses (304), Fitz gets her to give up the last of the bad batch, but only because he can trade them for other substances (307–08). Medical professionals should note the difference between the disciplinary inquiries of Fitz as opposed to Chen's student with addiction (312). Whereas Fitz protested "that his actions were justified, that he had only been prescribing you and many others what was needed" (312), the student "chose a wiser course—accepted responsibility for [her] portion of errors" (312). "Your issue," Chen writes to her, "was one of health, not professional conduct" (312). Yet she had been stealing from the pharmacy. Transgressions of professionals aren't tied to the behaviour itself so much as what story is told to explain it.

The most significant irony of Lam's book is that deaths are not allowed at Fitz's house, but someone dies during the clinical trial, suggesting that those operating outside the law rather than at the forefront of medical science are keeping people with addictions safer. When Chen asks what will happen to Fitz's users when his house is reappropriated, Fitz says "They'll find what they need, Chen, people always do" (339). The practitioner who has been pushed offside from the medical profession has the greatest clarity about the needs of patients with addictions. This devastating conclusion shows once more the intractable challenge that is Lam's primary focus throughout this book—the dilemmas of the opioid crisis and the torment of everyone, caregivers and sufferers alike, living on the brink of its ravine.

Depression: Miriam Toews's *All My Puny Sorrows* (2014)

All My Puny Sorrows is Miriam Toews's encounter with depression through a fictionalized account of the illness and suicide of her sister. The work follows Yoli as she tries to care for her sister Elf during her final months of hospitalization. In Toews's book Elf's piano playing reflects Claire's violin in Lam's, as music in both works offers a metaphor for an overburdened spirit suffering from mental illness. Caring often falls to family members, and beyond depression itself Toews's topic is the caregiving of family in contention with a medical profession that, in her telling, seems best at failing to care. Toews chronicles friction with medical practitioners, the unequal treatment received by cardiac and psychiatric patients, and the desperation of family to ease their loved one's suffering.

Toews examines how the blame suffered by those with mental illnesses adds to their burden. Yoli is constantly striving for greater empathy for her sister, observing the innocence of them both, along with other family members (181). Everyone suffers, is vulnerable, and mental illness is an equalizing force. "You haven't done anything bad or wrong," Janice, one of the few understanding nurses says to Elf. "You've acted on a feeling. Right? You wanted to end your suffering" (23). The need to remove blame and guilt from the healing process shows the extent to which patients suffering from suicidal ideation are burdened with the moral judgments of others. Towards the end of the novel Yoli tells her sister "that I understood that pain is sometimes psychic, not only physical" (246), a revelation of the real nature of mental illness. When Elf apologizes to her uncle for being in the hospital, in Yoli's telling, "He said no. We don't apologize for being sick, for being human, for being weary (Uncle Frank has obviously never been a woman)" (239). While Toews is pointing to gender differences in feelings of guilt, the observation that everyone suffering as a result of Elf's depression is innocent, including Elf herself, speaks to the stigma and blame associated with mental illness.

Toews contrasts differences in care and interpretation between Elf's depression and the cardiac illnesses her mother and aunt experience. Seeking ways to differentiate between illnesses of the heart and mind, Yoli muses that "A heart attack comes from the pain of remembering. . . . Or does a heart attack come from clogged arteries and fat around the waist and a two-pack-a-day habit and trans fats, not memories of pain and horror and unbearable sorrow?" (181). Mental and physical suffering can seem similar, yet the two forms of ailment are diagnosed very differently. When her aunt is hospitalized suddenly, the nurse can answer Yoli's questions about her coronary trouble (182). Diagnosing cardiac trouble is much simpler than explaining the origins of mental illness. Medical imaging and blood tests can provide clear answers for internal medicine, a diagnostic simplicity that seems to put practitioners at ease. At Yoli's aunt's bedside, "The nurse laughed and squeezed my arm. Nurses in cardio are far more playful and friendly than they are in psych" (219), Yoli observes, concluding that "If you have to end up in the hospital, try to focus all your pain in your heart rather than in your head" (219). Because she has two family members simultaneously hospitalized for cardiac and mental illness, the differences in care between the two ailments are stark to Yoli. In Toronto, when her mother has a cardiac event (307–8), Yoli observes that "hers was a cardio case not a head case so there were no lectures from the staff, no righteous psych nurse demanding of her: why won't you behave?" (308). Rather than having a single standard of care among different kinds of ailments, this book observes the denigration faced by those suffering from mental illness.

Yoli's family also resists medical care. She writes that "The experts involved had the hardest time understanding our family's extreme hostility to the entire health network. *We* had the hardest time understanding our family's extreme hostility to the entire health network" (50). Despite their lack of interest in engaging with the profession, because of their family history of depression, they are continually forced to interact with health workers: "How many times would I beg hospitals not to let my people go?" Yoli asks, explaining how she and her sister had "begged and begged and begged" to have their father kept in hospital to avoid his death by suicide, to no avail (225). "We are only family," she says. "And the doctors are busy packing as many appointments into a day as they can to pay for the next cycling holiday in the Pyrenees" (225). Being "only family" prevents them from being able to sway decision-makers. Yoli explains that she and her brother-in-law "are approaching the task of caring for Elf from two entirely different angles, from a sterile laboratory and from the dark side of the moon" (95). Whereas "He is pragmatic, scientific, and believes in prescriptions, in doctors' orders and in their omnipotence" (95), Yoli's most vivid concept of collaborating with doctors comes from the idea of getting one to "knock her out for good" by illegally giving her sister life-ending medication:

> we could find a doctor willing to bust into a hospital stash and steal them? Or maybe it's not even stealing if a doctor takes them. Call of duty. Or a willing pharmacist? Maybe a gang. There are a thousand gangsters in Winnipeg with access to illegal drugs. Or guns.
>
> *(151)*

This reference to interfaces between the illicit drug trade and hospital provenance of medication recalls *On the Ravine* and represents two kinds of usually parallel administration for dispensing drugs.

Caring for Elf is a collaboration between her family and the hospital workers, one that does not always satisfy either group. They often disagree over what she most needs. For example, Yoli relates how "The nurse who was not Janice was telling my mom that she agreed with her, Elf was a human being, but that she was also a patient in the hospital and was expected to cooperate," to which their mother demands to know why, and

> What does co-operation have to do with her getting well? Is co-operation even a symptom of mental health or just something you need from the patients to be able to control every last damn person here with medication and browbeating?
>
> *(214)*

While the healthcare providers have particular desires for model patient behaviour, family priorities emphasize a different approach to her overall well-being.

The greatest gap between these sets of expectations comes in the decision-making process around Elf's fatal hospital release. Elf needs a team of caregivers in place before she's safe to be released from hospital (49) and hospital staff make multiple promises not to let Elf leave (224, 247). One nurse repeatedly says that the question of her departure is "for the doctor to decide" (247), yet he "is never available to talk" (257). Yoli's favourite nurse reassures her about Elf by saying "We promise we won't let her go home until we have follow-up care in place" (248). But, called home to Toronto by her daughter's need (254), Yoli isn't able to keep watching over Elf: she's released and dies (261–62). Reflecting the torment of impossible prioritization facing many caregivers, Elf seizes the opportunity created by Yoli's obligations to her daughter. Just as in *Obasan*, where a mother's departure to care for her grandmother leaves a child without her mother's care (64), the stretching of Yoli's devotion between her sister and daughter, the question of how she can choose one's need over the other's, is a source of trouble in the narrative that permits Elf's death. Toews dramatizes the stretch here in the span of Canada's broad geography. Toronto and Winnipeg are perhaps not far psychologically, but they are separated by a major distance in practice. Elf's death happens because of two devastating and intractable gaps in care: between Yoli's and the hospital's view of her needs, and between Yoli's care for her daughter and sister at once.

A terrible psychiatrist sharpens Yoli's view of what kind of care she does want for her sister. While Elf is refusing to speak, he visits for the first time but will not take time to communicate with her through writing (174). In response to Yoli's complaint that he's not engaging with her sister's care, he says, "You're not the first family member to take out your frustration on me" (175). She shouts after him as he leaves, "if you won't help her then who will?" (175). This desperate plea calls into question what real help might look like. Later when Yoli asks a nurse for an update about Elf, she's unhelpfully told to ask the doctor (183). The experience as a whole pushes Yoli to articulate her understanding of care that could be helpful, asking the reader to "Imagine a psychiatrist sitting down with a broken human being saying, I am here for you. . . . You are experiencing great pain right now and it is my job and my mission to cure you from your pain" (176). Yoli's description of better care draws attention to how emotional support can be therapeutic, that medicine may be beneficial partly because of the relationship between the caregiver and patient. Yet psychiatrists are not always trained to offer the support Yoli wants, and the profession tends to be geared towards medication rather than the more talk-oriented treatments offered by other kinds of therapists (Scull 379), though some are looking to change this state of affairs (Novais et al.). As she imagines a doctor phoning late at night with updates, Yoli ultimately decides that "I won't give up on you" is what patients and their families most need to hear from physicians (177). Again and again Toews points out a paucity of care from the medical system in the face of mental illness. Beyond failures of sympathy alone, Toews's story critiques systems of medical training and administration that leave Yoli and her family craving more care than their providers have been equipped to offer.

Throughout the book, euthanasia represents a possibly viable and less painful alternative to suicide. Yoli's old philosophy professor "was on CBC panels all the time, talking about euthanasia, about all sorts of things having to do with the right to die, basically" (221). Elf herself asks Yoli to bring her to Switzerland to access assisted death (88, 90). Their mother however "made an executive decision" (245) and provided the service to their grandfather at the end of his life (245). After he'd been bedridden for nine years, their uncle tells Yoli, "Thankfully your mother pulled the plug when she did. Well, not literally pulled the plug, but one day she just decided to let him die" (244). Despite her training as a nurse, "She didn't suction him," so "His lungs filled up with fluid and she held his hand and said the things we say in times like that and let him go. Best thing she could have done for him" (245). This story of a passively assisted death puts forward a noteworthy end-of-life scenario in this book that ruminates about euthanasia. Though she contemplates the plan, however, Yoli cannot go through with it for her sister, writing, "You knew I didn't have the guts to take you to Zurich didn't you?" (318). Published before Canada officially sanctioned medical assistance in dying in 2016, or considered opening the service to those with mental illness, Toews's book offers an important consideration of the issue within a Canadian context.

Like Toews herself, Yoli is also a writer, and readers should attend to the meaning of reading, writing, and poetic interpretations of suffering in this text, a literary perspective that also opens moments of irony and gallows humour. While Yoli references Goethe on suicide (278), Elf recites the Philip Larkin poem "Days" to a pastor who makes an unwanted visit (224). In Larkin's poem answering the question of where can we live except in days, "Brings the priest and the doctor/In their long coats/Running over the fields" (qtd. in Toews 224). While Elf's ironic choice of poem reflects her situation, subject to doctors and priests, this literary treatment of time also chimes throughout the book. Yoli says that Elf "was a subject like time in that I couldn't grasp it but it had a mighty hold on *me*" (52). Of having the crushed possessions of her father returned to them after his death by suicide, Yoli writes, "His watch too. Time. Smash it. His wedding rings were bashed and nearly all of his two hundred and six bones broken" (48). The title of the book references a Coleridge poem Toews quotes: "I too a SISTER had, an only Sister—/She lov'd me dearly, and I doted on her!/ To her I pour'd forth all my puny sorrows/(As a sick Patient in his Nurse's arms)" (237). This quotation references not only grief but the scene of care between a sick patient and a nurse mapped onto a relation with a sister that is also the subject of this book. Though Elf is devoted to literature, her own writing has been reduced to one word, as Yoli observes that "I looked at her notebook and saw the word *pain* written at least fifty times. I picked it up. Shopping list? I said" (239). In another instance of Toews's dark and literary humour, when a child starts eating his grandmother's ashes during his mother's eulogy, Yoli observes that "just because someone is eating the ashes of your protagonist doesn't mean you stop telling the story" (254). Toews presents this scene with morbid comedy, but the moment also expresses Yoli's own compulsion to narrate the story despite the immense destruction and loss she faces. Such moments when the story seems to comment on itself produce the gentle self-consciousness of this novel that is, according to one commentator, a work of autofiction (see Reed 10–11). Throughout, Toews uses reading, writing, and storytelling to draw attention to the status of her text as a literary representation.

Yoli is the writer of the family, and the book itself makes numerous literary references, but it is Elf and the sisters' father who exhibit the greatest craving for literature. Writing of her two family members with depression, Yoli explains that "It was my father and my sister who constantly beseeched my mother and me to read more, to find succour for life in books, to soothe our aches and pains with words and more words" (90). Libraries are of particular relevance to Elf. Yoli asks her, "But what *is* the bedrock of civilized society? Libraries, said Elf" (79). When Elf escapes supervision, it's through the pretence of having her husband visit the library for her, and Yoli thinks,

> Well, Elf, I thought, you're so clever. Getting him to leave you alone on the pretext of getting books. Of going to the library. Of course he'd do it. Books are what save us. Books are what don't save us. *(267)*

When she regards the stack of books Elf's husband borrowed for her, Yoli sees that "they had failed" (266). She recollects why her sister had insisted that libraries represented the best in civilization because of how borrowers promise to return books (267): "What other institution operates in such good faith, Yo?" (267). Though Toews leaves the comparison to ring on its own, readers should connect this conclusion to the broken promise of the hospital caring for Elf, which released her to death and failed to return her. Toews is questioning and comparing the intent and value of these two forms of public institution, the hospital and the library. Ideally both institutions trade on faith in the release of books or patients into the world with the hope that they will return as needed: permanent hospitalization or institutionalization results without this faith in return or hope for a cure—the forever restricted circulation of a non-lending library.

In the face of intractable mental illness, Yoli circles the idea of solutions and cures, and searches for appropriate responses to illness and loss, finding that relinquishing the hospital is part of her grieving process. In trying to understand her sister's treatment, Yoli writes

> Finally I asked Janice about the pills. I asked her what was in them. What was the active ingredient? Do they give her the impression that there is meaning to life or do they flatten her to the point where she doesn't care if there is or isn't?
>
> *(92)*

The complexity of mental illness provokes desires for clear chemical cures that also answer metaphysical questions. Struggling with her loss, Yoli keeps prank-calling her sister's hospital, asking to speak with Elf though she has died (295). Her mother knows of this habit, and when she herself is hospitalized, she tells Yoli to stop drinking and calling the hospital (312). Putting an explanation for the behaviour into words, "She asked me if I was trying to haunt the hospital" (313). This idea that a grieving family member might herself haunt her loved one's hospital room in retaliation against healthcare providers she views as responsible reflects a stark depiction of mourning. Yoli's mother points out that "the pain of letting go of grief is just as painful or even more painful than the grief itself" (314). She is just another of Toews's more or less effective caregivers who strive to connect and console. "It's not me who's survived," Yoli says, "who's picked up and gone on, who's saved my mother by bringing her to Toronto, it's my mother . . . and she's taken me with her" (292). Though Yoli has moved them both to Toronto, her elderly mother, herself in mourning, shows her the path to healing. As her mother dreams of frozen food during an overnight sleep clinic, Yoli realizes she "was dreaming of survival," and decides, "I wouldn't tell her that frozen foods are full of sulphates, who cares, when she was deep into the cure" (293). For these characters suffering from the many losses of mental illness, being deep into the cure means finding a way to endure.

Conclusion

Perhaps more than other conditions, mental affliction defies language, both for the ill, but also for those trying to understand or write about what seems to be going wrong. Hazel Price offers a helpful exploration of the shifting verbal references that result in her recent study of the changing language for mental illness in the press. Even the most common terminology used to point to this area of struggle often fails to offer a direct reference to it: "mental health" is sometimes used as a stand-in for mental illness, and the term "mental health illness" is gaining currency in popular media, representing a contradictory verbal paradox that captures the strenuous difficulty of talking both for and about unwell minds. Even as the literature discussed in this chapter helps to illuminate a literary history of medical assistance in dying in Canada, it also grapples with these communication challenges, as we have seen in Brown's depiction of his son's disability, in Lam and Bydlowska's stories of addiction, and in Toews's narrative of depression.

The challenge to verbal communication posed by mental anguish in these often-autobiographical works reflects one of the most common features of this genre of narrative art, which often thus questions the seeming transparency of writing as a medium and its ability to offer a precise window on real experiences (see Smith and Watson 201). As these works show, telling the story of mental suffering often forces storytellers to foreground the conditions of narration itself.

Through the examples of these diverse works treating mental affliction in Canada, we've seen intractable mental anguish and brutal failures of language, whether in connecting loved ones or expressing the feelings of those trying to assuage and understand illness. These works belong to a category of literature that Amelia DeFalco describes as using the particularity of subjective narration to convey "the ethical quandaries arising from attempts to respond to the needs of others" (8). In the hands of the authors discussed here, the effort to encounter and verbalize mental ailment often becomes an account of caregivers' struggles to preserve another's well being or to relay their own misery at their failure and fear of loss. In telling stories of their loved ones' suffering, these characters find they must speak of their own.

Works Cited

Avrahami, Einat. *The Invading Body: Reading Illness Autobiographies*. U of Virginia P, 2007.

Birney, Earle. "David." 1942. *Open Country*, edited by Robert Lecker, Nelson, 2008, pp. 274–80.

Brown, Ian. *The Boy in the Moon*. St. Martin's, 2009.

Brown, Ian. "L'Arche Co-Founder Jean Vanier Sexually Abused at Least 25 Women over Seven Decades, Report Finds." *The Globe and Mail*, 31 Jan. 2023, p. A5.

Brown, Ian. "Two Metres and a World Apart: Life in Lockdown for Me and My Disabled Son." *The Globe and Mail*, 9 May 2020.

Bydlowska, Jowita. *Drunk Mom: A Memoir*. Doubleday, 2013.

CAMH. "Medical Assistance in Dying (MAiD) and Mental Illness—FAQs." *The Centre for Addiction and Mental Health (CAMH)*, www.camh.ca/en/camh-news-and-stories/maid-and-mental-illness-faqs. Accessed 24 July 2024.

Couser, G. T. *Signifying Bodies: Disability in Contemporary Life Writing*. U of Michigan P, 2010.

DeFalco, Amelia. *Imagining Care: Responsibility, Dependency, and Canadian Literature*. U of Toronto P, 2016.

Drewniak, Dagmara. "'This Has Been a Painful Story to Tell': Excavating Stories of Motherhood, Alcohol Abuse, and Writing in Two North American Memoirs: *Lit* by Mary Karr and *Drunk Mom* by Jowita Bydlowska." *A/B: Auto/Biography Studies*, vol. 34, no. 2, May 2019, pp. 197–210.
Duffin, Jacalyn. *History of Medicine: A Scandalously Short Introduction.* 3rd ed., U of Toronto P, 2021.
Engel, Howard. *The Man Who Forgot How to Read.* HarperCollins, 2007.
Frank, Arthur W. *The Wounded Storyteller.* U of Chicago P, 1995.
Fuller, Danielle. "The Crest of the Wave: Reading the Success Story of Bestsellers." *Studies in Canadian Literature*, vol. 33, no. 2, 2008, pp. 40–59.
Gammel, Irene. "Reading to Heal: Anne of Green Gables as Bibliotherapy." *Anne's World: A New Century of Anne of Green Gables*, edited by Irene Gammel and Benjamin Lefebvre, U of Toronto P, 2010, pp. 82–99.
Goldman, Marlene. *Forgotten: Narratives of Age-Related Dementia and Alzheimer's Disease in Canada.* McGill-Queen's, 2017.
Hawkins, Anne Hunsaker. *Reconstructing Illness: Studies in Pathography.* Purdue UP, 1993.
Health Canada. *Advice to the Profession: Medical Assistance in Dying (MAID)*, 27 Mar. 2023, www.canada.ca/en/health-canada/services/publications/health-system-services/advice-profession-medical-assistance-dying.html.
Hofsess, John. "I Helped Eight People End Their Lives. By the Time You Read This, I'll Have Ended Mine." *Toronto Life*, 29 Feb. 2016.
Johnston, Ann Dowsett. *Drink: The Intimate Relationship Between Women and Alcohol.* HarperCollins Canada, 2013.
Kirkup, Kristy. "Ottawa to Seek Extension on Implementing Medical Assistance in Dying for Mental Illnesses." *The Globe and Mail*, 29 Jan. 2024.
Lam, Vincent. *On the Ravine.* Knopf, 2023.
Laurence, Margaret. *The Stone Angel.* McClelland & Stewart, 1964.
Lousley, Cheryl. "After Extraction: Idling in the Ruins in Michael Winter's and Alistair MacLeod's Neoliberal Fictions." *Studies in Canadian Literature*, vol. 45, no. 2, 2020, pp. 229–53.
MacLeod, Alistair. *No Great Mischief.* McClelland & Stewart, 1999.
Mistry, Rohinton. *Family Matters.* McClelland & Stewart, 2002.
Monet, Jacques. "Georges Vanier." *The Canadian Encyclopedia*, Historica Canada, 2018.
Munro, Alice. "The Bear Came Over the Mountain." *Hateship, Friendship, Courtship, Loveship, Marriage*, McClelland & Stewart, 2001, pp. 275–323.
Munsch, Robert. "All about Robert Munsch." *The Official Robert Munsch Site*, https://robertmunsch.com/about. Accessed 29 July 2024.
Novais, Filipa, et al. "Communication Skills in Psychiatry for Undergraduate Students: A Scoping Review." *Frontiers in Psychiatry*, vol. 13, Aug. 2022.
Polley, Sarah. *Run towards the Danger.* Penguin, 2022.
Price, Hazel. *The Language of Mental Illness: Corpus Linguistics and the Construction of Mental Illness in the Press.* Cambridge UP, 2022.
Purdy, Al. "Earle Birney." *Quarry*, vol. 44, no. 4, 1996, pp. 98–106.
Purdy, Al. "The Man Who Killed David." *Weekend Magazine* [*Globe and Mail*, Toronto], 14 Dec. 1974.
Reed, Sabrina. *Lives Lived, Lives Imagined: Landscapes of Resilience in the Work of Miriam Toews.* U of Manitoba P, 2022.
Reid, Lesley W., et al. "Ecstasy and Gateway Drugs: Initiating the Use of Ecstasy and Other Drugs." *Annals of Epidemiology*, vol. 17, no. 1, Jan. 2007, pp. 74–80.
Richler, Mordecai. *Barney's Version.* Knopf, 1997.

Row, Nan, et al. "Robert Munsch Reveals Battle with Addiction." *Global News*, 17 May 2010.

Rushton, Amy. "A Bubble in the Vein: Suicide, Community, and the Rejection of Neoliberalism in Hanya Yanagihara's *A Little Life* and Miriam Toews's *All My Puny Sorrows*." *World Literature, Neoliberalism, and the Culture of Discontent*, edited by Sharae Deckard and Stephen Shapiro, Springer, 2019, pp. 195–213.

Scholastic Canada. *Robert Munsch: All about Munsch*, www.scholastic.ca/munsch/biography.php. Accessed 29 July 2024.

Scull, Andrew. *Desperate Remedies: Psychiatry's Desperate Quest to Cure Mental Illness*. Belknap, 2022.

Smith, Sidonie, and Julia Watson. *Reading Autobiography: A Guide for Interpreting Life Narratives*. 2nd ed., U of Minnesota P, 2010.

Smith, Stephen. "The Life of Margaret Laurence." *Quill and Quire*, 27 Feb. 2004.

Sullivan, Rosemary. *Shadow Maker: The Life of Gwendolyn MacEwen*. HarperCollins, 1995.

Tait, Carrie, and Erin Anderssen. "Judge Pauses MAID Death as Father, Daughter Continue Court Fight." *The Globe and Mail*, 25 Mar. 2024.

Toews, Miriam. *All My Puny Sorrows*. 2014. Vintage, 2015.

Vickers, Neil. "Illness Narratives." *A History of English Autobiography*, edited by Adam Smyth, Cambridge UP, 2016, pp. 388–401.

4

REPRODUCTIVE TROUBLE

Maternal Health and Houses in Iconic Fiction

Pregnancy is not a disease, yet it does impact women's health. Like an illness, it represents a shift in stasis for women's lives and identities that parallels how it alters their bodies. This change in physical and emotional equilibrium offers a source of narrative and reflects the transformations in character that works of fiction about illness frequently chart. As this chapter explores, some of the most famous and influential works of Canadian fiction ever published circle pregnancy and maternal health, often using the house and home as spatial symbols for the physical disruptions of childbirth.

Beginning with Sinclair Ross's prairie classic *As For Me and My House* (1941), and moving to later twentieth-century works by three of Canada's most historically celebrated authors, Margaret Laurence, Alice Munro, and Margaret Atwood, this chapter next considers historical novels about midwifery by Ami McKay and Lawrence Hill, and closes with Sheila Heti's *Motherhood* (2018). Through these texts, the role of the midwife or doctor takes on a special status, while the house is often posed as a stand-in or counterpart to the womb as a space of mothering and the site of reproductive trouble.

Literary Celebrity and Maternal Health in Canada

Since many works that stand as classic touchstones within the Canadian canon concern maternal health, this chapter examines works that have been especially privileged in popular consciousness. A current that runs alongside this focus is the increasing twentieth-century publication and

DOI: 10.4324/9781003340119-5

celebration of books by women in Canada. Patricia Demers documents this history and spotlights the dominance of two literary celebrities, Alice Munro and Margaret Atwood, in late-twentieth- and early twenty-first-century notions of Canadian literature on an international stage, a context that Lorraine York explores in her study, *Literary Celebrity in Canada* (2007). This chapter examines the major impact of Munro and Atwood along with other highly celebrated authors through their depictions of reproductive health.

Atwood and Munro published the texts under consideration in this chapter in the 1970s and 1980s, but their lasting international stature is evident in their continued discussion in contemporary culture. While critics of Republican attacks on reproductive rights in the lead-up to the 2024 American election often referenced Atwood's Gilead (see Lederman, for example), the news in July 2024 that Munro failed to respond to her daughter's sexual abuse by her husband (Skinner) prompted an outpouring of questioning regarding the meaning of reading her work. Reacting in *The Cut* a day later, critic Michelle Dean suggested, "I know these stories better now than I did before because of this revelation." The question of how readers should respond to these discoveries touches on a long-standing concern in literary theory regarding whether and how authorial biography and intention matters when reading literature. This discussion draws on famous 1960s essays by Roland Barthes ("Death of the Author") and Michel Foucault ("What is an Author?") that question the significance of authors and their lives to the work of interpretation. The "Me Too" movement to publicize sexual abuses by prominent mostly male creators and advocate against the celebration of their work puts these questions newly into contention in the 2010s and 2020s (Jestrovic 25–26). Conversations are ongoing regarding how Munro's story fits into this realm of theory regarding reading the work of imperfect people and the extent to which parallels from authors' lives can be used to interpret their texts. For both Atwood and Munro, their ongoing relevance in contemporary conversations sustains their status as highly known figures in popular consciousness.

Sexual politics inform current concepts of both Atwood and Munro as literary celebrities, but maternal health is also an implicit if not always overt focus in the works of many other famous Canadian authors. For example, in an iconic scene, Dunstable Ramsay ducks a snowball at the beginning of Robertson Davies's *Fifth Business* (1970), letting it hit a pregnant woman and thus induce her labour early. The premature baby experiences lifelong ill health, leaving Ramsay with a guilt that drives the rest of the novel. Even as this work is propelled by a woman's traumatic experience of childbirth, the main agents and speaking characters are men. While Cynthia Sugars examines Davies's analogy between literary criticism and medicine in *The Cunning Man* (1994), Marlene Goldman explains that *Fifth Business* reflects a historic notion of hysteria as a mental illness associated with women and afflictions of the womb in the nineteenth and early twentieth centuries. Though it lost the 1970 Governor General's award to Dave Godfrey's now rarely read *The New Ancestors* (1970) (Mount, *Arrival* 38), Davies's book was often assigned in Canadian high schools, placing its strange focus on pregnancy as a source of narrative trouble as the first and sometimes only Canadian novel introduced to students during their public education.

Given this status as possibly one of the few novels read by many Canadian doctors, Davies's story may have had an outsized impact on how they view their roles, a hypothesis supported by two articles published nearly thirty years apart by Nova Scotia physician Ian A. Cameron (see "Observations" and "Family"). In contrast and published the same year as Davies's novel, Audrey Thomas's autobiographical and avant-garde account of miscarriage in *Mrs. Blood* (1970) let her write "about her own suffering" (Coldwell 46) and is far less known.

In another example of the widespread but not always acknowledged impact of disordered pregnancy in Canadian literature, one of the most popular Canadian books ever published with more than thirty-seven million copies sold (Firefly), Robert Munsch's children's story *Love You Forever* (1986) was written partly in mourning for his wife's two stillbirths (Munsch, "All about"). This context should inform interpretations of the strangely affecting scenes it portrays of a mother rocking her son at night even as he advances through the ages of life beyond when such care is welcome: the mother's maturing son only permits this cradling because he is lost in the oblivion of sleep, a counterpart to death itself, while her rocking is a gesture of mourning as well as love, and her own ageing signals the lifelong endurance of grief.

As efforts to combat the silence around pregnancy loss increase worldwide (WHO), the truth is that, sometimes more than they realize, Canadians have long told, celebrated, and been impacted by stories of troubled pregnancy, premature delivery, miscarriage, and stillbirth.

Sinclair Ross's *As For Me and My House* (1941)

Sinclair Ross's *As For Me and My House* (1941) considers how a stillbirth changes a woman's life and character. The novel cycles through Mrs. Bentley's experiences of adoption, until her final chance to mother a newborn occurs with the death of her husband's lover in childbirth. Though written by a male author, Ross's novel charts the first-person perspective of a woman whose tense and focused view of her world has captivated generations of readers. As the critic David Stouck suggests, the novel is full of "gaps and omissions that force the reader to take part in constructing the book's meaning," and as such it represents "one of Canada's first modernist works of fiction" ("Introduction" 3). This leveraging of silence to communicate indicates the modernity of Ross's novel, but these meaningful omissions and implications can also be read via the logic of gossip and the hint, which often use indirection to convey illicit detail.

Ross constructs Mrs. Bentley as a deeply conflicted soul whose desires for maternity sometimes seem subordinate to her love for her husband. The speaker describes herself as a "broodless old woman" (7), a description that reflects the persistent irony of Ross's style, since the speaker is only in her thirties (22), and, though she is "broodless," since she hasn't borne a living child, she is brooding—a doubly meaningful term that best reflects her ongoing ruminations. Like a broody hen, who falls into a kind of trance as she submits to a compulsion to sit on her eggs until they hatch, Ross's narrator dwells on and broods over the prospect of maternity.

As Ross's title indicates, the space of the house represents a key symbol throughout the book. Mrs. Bentley's husband, a minister, keeps changing posts, as towns tire of the couple (14), so they move every few years to another small prairie town made up of buildings with false fronts, and Mrs. Bentley describes putting up a false front of her own (13). Ross draws this connection between buildings and selfhood in his circling of the meaning of the house in Mrs. Bentley's life. The text her husband always uses for his first sermon in a new town is "As for Me and My House We Will Serve the Lord" (7). The couple uses the line for a sign outside their house announcing "the house of Bentley," a sign that hides, Mrs. Bentley suggests, "a tough, deep-rooted tangle" (81). More than a theme from Scripture, the trouble of the Bentleys' house is indicated by the disrepair of the home they have moved to in Horizon. Mrs. Bentley is depressed by the failures of the house, which leaks (8, 10). She feels its silence is hostile (77), while her discovery of a tobacco pipe (19) gives her a sense of its prior inhabitants. The pipe owner clearly also bent the pious rules of behaviour expected of ministers' families, giving Mrs. Bentley "the thought that we aren't the only ones" who didn't fully conform to religious expectations (20). Mrs. Bentley is both soothed and bothered by the evidence of past inhabitants in her house, just as Atwood's handmaiden finds reassurance and dismay in the traces left by her room's previous occupants, as we will later see. The "insistent" smell of the house, its "exhalation of the past," Mrs. Bentley writes, communicated "that this is a house of silence and repression and restraint" and "that its past will not be mocked" (77). Beyond the disrepair of their home, and the feeling of the presence of its prior residents, the couple's relationship also causes the disorder of their dwelling. Mrs. Bentley suggests that being alone in a house with just one other person is "difficult," and that "Every clink of a dish or fork is solitary and foreboding like a chip off the crack of doom" (21). To the extent that the Bentleys' lives are troubled, are in some way "bent," the house localizes and frames the disorder.

Ross focuses the disturbance within the house and within their family above all on their lack of a child and Mrs. Bentley's desperate effort to secure her husband's attention. This childlessness is a pathology, a sickness, that troubles the narrative. An artist with an "urge to create" (43), Philip's career as a minister has frustrated his aspirations, though "He still draws, cold little ghosts of his dream that are stronger than their uselessness" (45). Mrs. Bentley feels that if she had a son, she wouldn't have "wasted" his potential, just "postponed to another generation his fulfillment" (7). She describes their union with a resignation that also responds to their experience of reproduction: "Anyway, we were married. The next year there was a baby, stillborn" (45). The devastation of this loss prompts Philip to work on a book for the next year, rather than his visual art (59), as though the physicality of a book, roughly newborn-sized, could compensate for the missing infant. The book "was a failure" (84). He craves a son, which Mrs. Bentley observes in how he watches twelve-year-old twin boys, and imagines educating them, as, she writes, "he has a way of building in his own image" (9). Mrs. Bentley positions her husband's desire for a son as a replacement or replication of his desire to create. Mrs. Bentley dwells on the twelve years since the stillbirth, reflecting that "It takes twelve years without a boy to let you know how much one's worth" (216). She views herself as "a hindrance" (44) to him and suggests that she "kept him in the church" for twelve years (141), regrets stopping him from getting fired twelve years before (96), though "Comfort and routine were the last things he needed" (135). The job conflicts with his sense of himself as an artist, and Mrs. Bentley describes how "The constant sense of deceit and hypocrisy has been a virus, destroying his will and sapping his energy" (88). While their lifestyle has been a kind of sickness for him, she also compares herself to a "fungus or parasite whose life depends on his" (199). While as a couple they suffer from infertility, a pathology Mrs. Bentley blames on herself, she also describes Philip as beset by physical maladies of which she is the source of infection. She concludes that "He ought to have had the opportunity to live, to be . . . anything but what he is, what I've made him" (136), which reflects a repetition of the idea of creation that is tied up in their tortured relationship. She says that all she wants is to be noticed by him (23), and, in a twisted replacement of desire, she craves a son in the hopes of securing his attention at last.

Adoption offers the couple a way out of the childlessness that has soured their relationship. The first time, they take in a boy, Steve, who is in need of a home. Mrs. Bentley, a classically trained pianist, feels tender towards him, and describes the experience as a rediscovery as a piece of music that had been playing inside her unheeded for twelve years, that is, since her baby was born (91). The arrival of boy, "a son," also enlivens Philip (67), but the child quickly becomes a pawn in the Bentleys' unhappy relationship. Philip takes Steve to the country, partly for three "sick calls," but Mrs. Bentley "could feel that he didn't want me along, so at noon I complained of a headache" (60), but then she admits that "maybe I was expecting to hear him say the drive would do me good, or that he'd better put his visits off until another time" (60). She uses feigned illness to try to secure greater attention or commitment from her husband over their adopted child, but is once again thwarted. In retaliation, she plays the piano "vindictively," enrapturing Steve, to show Philip how "I could take the boy away from him" (63). While Mrs. Bentley is sure her husband doesn't understand Steve's character (70), she still envies their bond: realizing Philip has never needed her (84), when he drives off with Steve again, she sees "the worth of what I've always called a victory" (85). Steve experiences multiple conflicts with other boys in the town, which some scornfully blame on his biological parentage, though Mrs. Bird, the doctor's wife, says her husband "insists it's environment, not heredity" (79). Mrs. Bentley invokes Mark 2:17 in defense of Steve to judgmental women of the town, saying "it's the sick, isn't it, and not the whole" (81) who need the most care. Despite their efforts to keep and care for the boy, Catholic church officials take him (152) because the Bentleys are Protestants. Ross's depiction of this failed adoption underscores the infertility of this couple.

Ross implies that deficiency in the Bentleys' sex life might be responsible for their childlessness, and he both gestures toward sex and leaves it out. While conforming to norms regarding the elision of sex from literary depictions of this period, Ross does illustrate the couple's uncomfortable bed sharing. Philip frequently stays up waiting for Mrs. Bentley to be asleep before he goes to bed (148). When he does come to bed while she's awake, Ross often details their silent tension. Describing their wakefulness through the night, she senses "the strain of his rigid, aching muscles" and reaches out her hand to him, but "there was a sharp little contraction against my touch" and she pulls away again (153). Through this chronicling of what seems to be a mostly sexless marriage, occasionally Ross does imply physical consummation between the Bentleys, but always with a subtlety to suit censorious literary standards. For example, when it rains, the couple experiences a bit of romance, as the house seems to close around them,

> driven in by the night and wetness. He didn't speak, but I think he was glad of me again. He slept soon, and I lay a long time listening to the rain. It was good to have him to myself again.
>
> *(155)*

In such oblique references to their physical intimacy, Ross shows that the marriage isn't entirely sexless. Yet these instances frequently signal uncomfortable sex: Mrs. Bentley describes not pretending to be asleep one night when he comes to bed, and writes that "He didn't mind, but he wasn't eager either. Kind still, far off, as if he were sorry" and "felt it was the least he could do" (158). Sex as "the least he could do" reflects the weakness of their physical connection. Mrs. Bentley also describes the couple's sex after she learns of his affair: she notes that "Last night he didn't wait as usual for me to be asleep, and I was glad. . . . That's how much he means to me. I'll take him anyway" (166). She works to maintain their sexual relationship despite his faithlessness, yet the pursuit comes at a cost. She tries to interest him, bringing on her own self-loathing, until sometimes "The night comes when he wants me, but it brings no ease or sense of consummation," and leaves her awake and ashamed, "living again through the night I listened to him with her" (199). The antithesis of an erotic text, this book focalizes awkward moments in bed, as though offering proof of what's missing in this marriage in which childlessness is a pathology. The implication is that their core trouble of infertility might be solved if they had more—and better—sex.

The sex that does lead to procreation, however, occurs as the result of illness. Mrs. Bentley seems to be aware from the start of the growing partiality between her husband and Judith. She watches as "He met her glance, and for the first time I saw the whiteness of her face give way to a little flush of color" (73). Judith blushes again when Philip looks at her (94), then he blushes when she looks at him (94), and later she looks at him "admiringly" (142). All these flushed glances are seen through the eyes of Mrs. Bentley, as the book never strays from her first-person perspective. They should be read for the signalling of shame and desire Mary Ann O'Farrell illustrates in blushes in nineteenth-century novels. Catching sight of the outline of Judith's body as her clothes press against her in the wind makes Mrs. Bentley realize that "she had never occurred to me as a woman before," a category of person she's feared ever since meeting her husband (102). In retaliation for the attraction that she senses between them, she invites Judith to dinner "to watch her eyes follow him, her breathing quicken a little—to look then at him, and know how completely it was wasted" (144).

Mrs. Bentley's effort to manage her rival is rendered futile when she falls ill. She is so sick that she visits the doctor, who uses a stethoscope to listen to her chest, diagnoses neuritis, and prescribes bed rest (159). Despite these instructions, Mrs. Bentley explains that "bed is where I mustn't stay" (159), since she wants to avoid obliging her husband to care for her. Due to his misogynist revulsion at doing work prescribed for women, she says "I know it would rouse a loathing in him if he had to be my nurse" (159).

To avoid this outcome, Philip suggests that Judith come to care for Mrs. Bentley, who contends that "It will take a worse ache in my shoulder than this one to keep me in the bedroom while she sits out here alone with him" (160). Readers should note Ross's contrasting use of pain and pleasure through this episode. "For the nights Dr. Bird let them give me sleeping powders," Mrs. Bentley explains, but, while taking her dose one evening, she spills some, so that "there had just been enough of the powder to stupify" her (161). When she awakes and creeps from her room, it's the sound of laughter that alerts her to the illicit nature of what is happening in the lean-to where Judith is staying. She describes it as a laugh "that I've laughed often with him too. There's no other laugh like it" (162). The laughter here, involuntary, physical, pleasurable, is a stand-in for sex itself, and as Mrs. Bentley listens to it, she writes, "I just stood there listening a minute, a queer, doomed ache inside me" (162). While Mrs. Bentley was prescribed medication for pain that nearly blinded her to her husband's betrayal, witnessing the pleasure he gives another also causes her pain. Mrs. Bentley's illness makes room for her husband's infidelity, for rule-breaking sex. As I discuss shortly, echoes of this pattern recur in *Lives of Girls and Women*, when Del's experience with Mr. Chamberlain occurs because her friend is sick (152–59). While Mrs. Bentley's illness makes room for the adultery, the medication provides cover, and the failure of the dosage reveals the betrayal by letting Mrs. Bentley awake in time to discover it.

Ross represents the stakes of this adultery through a focus on the bed. Once more, when Philip returns to her bed at last, Mrs. Bentley pretends to sleep (163), replaying the usual outcome of their nights together. She realizes he's committed adultery, and that she could be free of him, but still can't be (163), and suggests his betrayal doesn't reveal particular affection for Judith, as though in a Shakespearean bed trick drama, bodies in sexual encounters may be swapped in for others: "Deep inside I even know that it really isn't Judith. She was just there. Another time somebody else will be there" (171). When she's first prescribed bed rest, Mrs. Bentley writes, "I wish it were Philip who had been ordered to his bed. I think it's what I've really been wishing ever since we met" (160). It is characteristic of Ross's variety of narrative irony that in the end it is Philip who does wind up in bed when he shouldn't be.

The news of Judith's pregnancy is relayed to Mrs. Bentley in conversation with the doctor's wife (192), showing the real porousness of presumed confidentiality between doctor and patient. The doctor also predicts the due date—"sometime in May" (192). Due to the medicalization of childbirth, doctors assume powerful roles in reproduction. During the pregnancy, Mrs. Bentley suffers through Christmas (a festival of birth), calling it "a bleak season in a childless home" (194), and saying that "It's worse this time because at last there is a child, and it isn't mine" (195). She compares the feeling to an "abscess" (195), once more confirming Ross's association between physical illnesses and the yearning for love, whether maternal or romantic. Anticipating "what's going to happen when the baby's born" (199), Mrs. Bentley sends Philip to see Judith (199) along with a vindictive gift of oranges, which make Judith cry "all afternoon, one in each hand" (201). In this strange image that invites a reading of the oranges as a visual stand-in for breasts, the untasted fruit represents the difficulty and joy of breastfeeding that Judith will never experience. Mrs. Bentley acknowledges the internal conflicts that drive the tension of her prose in announcing, "I've fought it out with myself and on at last. We're going to adopt Judith's baby" (202). Though she attacks Judith obliquely with the falsely sympathetic gift of oranges, the real struggle is with herself. Mrs. Bentley brings up her plan for the baby with Philip when they're in bed, saying "I've always liked Judith. Better than anyone else's I think I could take her baby and forget it isn't mine" (203–4). This scene replicates the earlier suggestion of bodies swapping in bed, and it is notable that the prospect of a child becomes real for the couple when they are in bed together, in a scene that positions a decision to adopt as located in the bed as much as sexual reproduction: babies come from couples being alone in bed together. Mrs. Bentley anticipates the birth with a fierce insistence that "I want it to be my baby—my son. I won't let her remind me that it isn't" (204). "Every day," she writes, "my nerves get sharper, tenser. My baby—his baby—all I have of him. It's going to be a boy, of course, and I'm going to call him Philip too" (207). The strange and intense perspective of this book becomes most acute during this period of gestation.

Mrs. Bentley is characteristically understated in relaying the key dramatic moment of the narrative: "Judith's baby was born Monday night, a month before its time. Judith died early Tuesday morning" (211). The baby's physical calamity at being born prematurely is quickly eclipsed by the death of his mother. Mrs. Bentley hears the news once again from the doctor's wife, who brings the baby to her, because the "doctor wanted him in town where he could watch him and see he was being fed properly" (211). The doctor again predicts and sanctions how the baby enters the community. In parenthood, Philip starts to look like the baby, with "a stillness, a freshness, a vacancy of beginning" (216), and the book closes with Mrs. Bentley's suggestion that in naming the baby Philip she will get her husband and son mixed up—her ultimate goal (216).

The novel resolves the pathology of Mrs. Bentley's childlessness through Judith's death in childbirth. That the conception occurs during Mrs. Bentley's own illness shows how Ross multiplies physical ailments, so that one character's illness eventually leads to another's postpartum death. The implication that Mrs. Bentley's constant goal has been to finally secure and replicate her husband and his love reveals another underlying pathology in this novel. The Oedipal suggestion that she aims to confuse her son and husband can be read as one of the sicknesses of love that, as Jacalyn Duffin establishes, literature since ancient Greece has often examined.

In encountering the elusive voice of this text written by a man and the strange story of desire it tells in a straight woman's perspective, it's important to note the potential for queer readings. The curious perspective of this book, so compelling to so many returning readers, may be interpreted as the queer gaze of a repressed, spurned lover on an idol who doesn't share the attraction, whose own attraction is to a childbearing woman. Indeed, critics often read this work through a queer lens (see Estok; Lesk), and among the stillbirths at the heart of this narrative may be unspoken desire and subsumed gender identification in the perspective of its narrator. Though he had sex with men, critics and historians have debated whether Ross himself identified as a gay man (C. Hill), a category that became clearer and more permissible through the course of the eighty-eight years between his birth in 1908 and death in 1996. In his biography *As For Sinclair Ross* (2005), David Stouck contends that the author preferred the "greater range" of bisexuality and that the dynamics of his single life with couples for friends are reflected in his fiction's "patterns of triangulated desire" (x). Indeed, rather than reflecting a romantic relationship in the author's own life, the household scene of *As For Me and My House* resembles his tense but relentless relationship with his mother, with whom he lived long into adulthood, and whose dominance he escaped in silence (Stouck, *As For* 29). Whatever models helped Ross imagine Mrs. Bentley, her perspective remains startlingly fresh and acute.

Because of its modern perspective and publication history, Ross's novel has had an outsized impact in Canadian letters. The author destroyed other novels he wrote that failed to sell, and this could easily have been the fate of *As For Me And My House* if not for a wealthy American's choice to publish it on first reading without concern for its commercial viability—which proved minimal (Stouck, "Introduction" 5–6). This history reflects Nick Mount's point in *When Canadian Literature Moved to New York* (2005), that the notion of Canadian literature has long been dependent on American publishers. Though the novel did not win the Governor General's Award for the year it was published, sixteen years later, in 1957, the editors starting the influential New Canadian Library series cemented its longevity in the Canadian canon by reissuing it as a paperback and hailing it as a "classic" (Stouck, "Introduction" 6). As a result, the powerful frustrations of Mrs. Bentley's experience as a wife became available for a younger generation of readers at a time when the wave of feminism of the 1960s and 1970s was gathering force. Ross's novel may never have enjoyed widespread popularity among a general readership, but its literary complexity and accomplishment places it in a Canadian category of its own for the period and ensures that it continues to be taught.

Margaret Laurence's "To Set Our House in Order" (1970)

If birth causes disorder in fiction, it is often a disorder of the house. Margaret Laurence's short story, "To Set Our House in Order," was first published in *The Ladies Home Journal* in 1964 and included in the author's influential collection *A Bird in the House* (1970). The narrative is a haunting meditation on a child's place in the home that erupts from the disorder caused by her mother's difficult pregnancy. Vanessa dwells over the extent to which she can stand in for her stillborn sister, while the role of physician lets her father stand in for his brother, even as he can't act as a doctor for his wife. The landscape of the home provides the stage for these swapping roles in a troubled clockwork whose disruptions and gaps reveal more chaos than order.

Vanessa initiates her first-person story with the discovery of a problem with her mother's pregnancy. "When the baby was almost ready to be born," the story begins, "something went wrong and my mother had to go into the hospital two weeks before the expected time" (39). The fact of having a story to tell, trouble to relay, derives from the dislocation of this experience: the child's feeling of wrongness results from her mother's departure, which itself results from her mother's physical ailment. The vagueness of this "something" that is wrong reflects a child's perspective on medical problems, since she may not have understood the issue, but was also unlikely to have been told what it was. In any case, the medical problem itself is irrelevant to a child: what matters is the removal of her mother from the home. The home is sent into disarray by the mother's departure to the hospital, which, though it is not a primary setting for this story, stands as the ghostly counterpart to the house. The rest of Laurence's story flows from this primary disruption.

The limitation of a child's perspective on illness and medical care is essential to this story. Her father is a doctor, and her sense of trouble is accentuated by listening to him make an anxious call to another doctor (39). She says,

> I believed him to be not only the best doctor in Manawaka, but also the best doctor in the whole of Manitoba if not in the entire world, and the fact that he was not the one who was looking after my mother seemed to have something sinister about it.
>
> *(41)*

The concept that a physician should not care for his family members is illogical for a child. While Vanessa experiences a dislocation in having her mother leave the home, seeing her father pass off her mother's care is another displacement for her. Throughout, the story foregrounds the disjunction between what children intuit or perceive and what they are invited to witness about birth and illness. Though Vanessa wants to visit her mother, she's told that "Kids aren't allowed to visit maternity patients" (49). A desire to prevent infection likely backs this rule, but it also contains a painful irony—that mothers can't see children while having more children. Without understanding or being told the medical rationale, for a child, only the irony and confusion of this rule are salient. Such uncomfortable contradictions between children and adults' perspectives on medical care recur throughout the story. When her father tells her about the operation her mother will have to remove the baby, "He kept on saying it was not serious nowadays" (50), in a repetition that seems more worrying than reassuring. When explaining to her why he would not be providing medical care to her mother, "he put on that difficult smile with which adults seek to conceal pain from children" (41). The idea of being familiar with such a particular smile reinforces how children may be acutely aware of the suffering of the adults around them, and the futility of their attempts at concealment.

Her grandmother's ailments also challenge Vanessa's capacity to understand. While her mother is in hospital because of her pregnancy, her grandmother suffers from headaches, and often lies in bed (43), just as Vanessa's mother does for weeks when she finally returns home with the baby (56). Vanessa's father attributes his mother's ailments to "troubles in her life," which are "why she gets migraine sometimes and has to go to bed" (53). Changed financial circumstances are part of her distress, but the primary aspect of these "troubles" is the loss of her son Rod. Having been blinded in one eye by Vanessa's father's air rifle (56), Rod hid his injury to join the army, only to die from battle wounds in his brother's arms (57). In a letter about his death to their mother, Vanessa's father wrote of his brother's gallantry, but told his wife later that "men don't really die like that" (57). Once more injuries multiply throughout the family, so the wound to Rod's eye seems to presage his death in battle, which itself renders his mother sometimes bedridden. More than the generational inheritance of a profession, it seems to be guilt that has sent Vanessa's father into the medical profession, as "It was only after the war that he decided to come back and study medicine and go into practice with his father" (58). Since Vanessa's mother never felt she could ask whether Rod would have also become doctor (58), Laurence implies that an effort to make up for the loss of his brother might have driven the choice.

Besides the loss of her son, her change in status also troubles Vanessa's grandmother. While Vanessa comes from a long line of people with doctors for fathers, the social and financial meaning of this position has changed a great deal through the course of the three generations the story regards. "[H]is father was a doctor," Vanessa's father says of his own father, "so that's what he was" (51), showing the often-paternal descent of the profession. Though she claims to have been born in a castle in Scotland, Vanessa's grandmother was born in Ontario and "father was a horse doctor" (49). She married a medical physician, though, and "He soon had more patients than either of the other doctors. We ordered our dinner service and all our silver from Birks in Toronto" (45). For her, being married to a doctor brought a sense of affluence and status to which she clings, despite massive economic changes. Although, as Vanessa's father says, "People can't entirely dispense with doctors or undertakers" (47), his patients are now paying their bills in chickens (47). Laurence's story is partly about how historical changes in the circumstances of doctors impact their wives.

This change in financial security bothers Vanessa's grandmother most and becomes visible in her effort to manage the household. She describes her early relationship with her husband, and his insistence that, despite living with him in rural places, she would have "a proper house" (45). She has a penchant for ordering expensive housewares from catalogues (48–49), while her desire to hire a housekeeper that the family can't afford causes tension with Vanessa's father (47), and she suggests that his wife's pregnancy wouldn't be troubled had he hired more help around the house (40). He explains to his daughter that "the house is still the same, so she thinks other things should be too" (53). The house itself is the scene of her efforts at dominion, but also the locus of her losses, both personal and financial.

For Vanessa too, the house takes on immense meaning. She lurks about while waiting for her brother to be born, and "spent the morning morbidly, in seeking hidden places in the house. There were many of these" (42). She doesn't want to go out to play, because she "had the feeling that if I left the house, even for a few hours, some disaster would overtake my mother" (42). For Vanessa, the house always seems full of sounds (41), and presences she knew belonged to

> every person, young or old, who had ever belonged to the house and had died, including Uncle Roderick who got killed on the Somme, and the baby who would have been my sister if only she had managed to come to life.
>
> *(42)*

The house locates the presence of the dead. In this mysteriously enchanted space, Vanessa is a kind of interloper. The house "never seemed like home" to her (43), and when her grandmother finds her dusty from the attic, she looks at her like a "cockroach that had just crawled impertinently out of the woodwork" (44). Resembling an insect's infiltration, the child's placement in this home is akin to wildlife in the landscape of the house.

The house is the primary scene of the disrupted order that this story also reflects in the troubled pregnancy. Before leaving for the hospital, Vanessa's mother promises that her grandmother will "keep everything in order, and then some" (40). Laurence links this desire for order to household management. "My accounts were always in good order," Vanessa's grandmother says, "and so was my house" (46). Drawing out the words that title the story, she explains to Vanessa that her own father always said, "God loves Order—he wants each one of us to set our house in order" (46). This phrase rings throughout the story, begging the question of what it means in a context where a bit of household help is proposed as a solution to every problem, from the maladies of pregnancy to the ravages of grief. The house itself gives a scene for all these troubles, and the prospect of order in the home seems to offer hope. Yet one outcome of dwelling for generations in the same house is the feeling of overlapping roles, like marionettes changing places in the same rooms. Once more grappling with the contradictions between the limited comprehension of a child and potent emotional sensitivity, Vanessa thinks about the dead baby "who might as easily have been I" (59), and her new living brother (59), who her grandmother demands be named for her dead son (55). While family members seem possibly able to stand in for each other, in dreams she "could hear the caught sparrow fluttering in the attic, and the sound of my mother crying, and the voices of the dead children" (53). The attic offers a space both within and without of the house, representing, like a bird caught in the wrong landscape, the feeling of trespass and overlap in living in spaces still somehow occupied by the dead. "A bird in the house means a death in the house," a character says in the story that gives this collection its title (102). This feeling of death at the heart of a living space is the ultimate sense of disorder that this story documents, as Vanessa closes the story, writing, "I could not really comprehend these things, but I sensed their strangeness, their disarray. I felt that whatever God might love in this world, it was certainly not order" (59). Laurence maps this sense of disorder to the space of the house.

In a haunting proliferation of the risks and traumas of motherhood, this story about illness in pregnancy repeats a narrative about a mother's loss of a child, both in the story of Vanessa's mother's stillbirth, and the story of Roderick's death in battle. Laurence proposes that the disorders and illnesses that her story chronicles, of love, of death, of birth, of money and inheritance, are problems of the house. Vanessa's mother's troubled pregnancy and birth, as well as her difficult medical history of stillbirth, prompt this narrative. Laurence places the elusive complexity of all these relationships within the space of the house, where feelings can be locked away like objects in attic storage, and voices of the dead still echo. In this domestic space, one person or baby can seem to substitute for another, as easily as trading a bedroom, or swapping places at the dinner table. Through these exchanges, the role of the doctor is as a witness and usher to birth and death, promising and withholding power over these metaphysical moments, while also representing a burden of professional care that characters may pass between each other and across generations.

Alice Munro's *Lives of Girls and Women* (1971)

By comparing the lives of several women at different life stages, Alice Munro's *Lives of Girls and Women* (1971) contrasts life options for women. Pregnancy, birth, and reproductive health are primary concerns of Del and the women she knows, while access to birth control impacts their sense of agency. The book can be read as examining and testing the veracity of the advice that Del describes as received wisdom, the idea that "being female made you damageable" (165). Sex and pregnancy are among the key concerns of this book, which scrutinizes how women permit and avoid these experiences, the danger of birth, and the justice and empowerment of reproductive control.

Through Del's eyes, the book dwells over illness, affliction, and death. Her Uncle Craig, blind in one eye (29), dies of heart attack (45), while her Auntie Grace stays in hospital "recovering, as it was thought, from a broken hip" (60), in an oblique hint, characteristic of Munro's style, that her real diagnosis may not have been disclosed. Del's cousin Mary Agnes touches a dead cow's eye (44), while Fern, who rooms with Del's family, questions whether mental illness among the children of Mrs. Sherriff results from the second generation impacts of a syphilis infection contracted by her husband (96). The librarian is "deaf as a stone and lame in one leg from polio," and the town has given her the job to accommodate her disability (111). "Your Uncle Bill is a dying man," Del's mother bursts out, to explain the sudden arrival of her brother (85), while the two of them discuss whether their mother died in pain or if anaesthetic helped her at the end (83). Del bites Mary Agnes hard enough to draw blood in retaliation for being forced to look at their dead uncle's body at his funeral (53), a move that results in invocations of the doctor, pills for Aunt Moira, and Del being put on the couch, "as if I was sick" (54). Del's mother is preoccupied by the possibility of organ donation in future (47), echoing the Metaphysical poet John Donne's famous sonnet, "Death be not Proud," in saying that death wouldn't then be a conversation topic because "We would all be heirs of one another's bodies, we would all be donors too. Death as we know it now would be done away with!" (47). This pervasive atmosphere of morbidity is part of Del's constantly thwarted desire to understand mortality: "I wanted death pinned down and isolated behind a wall of particular facts and circumstances, not floating around loose" (45). The epilogue opens with a focus on how the town is experiencing a wave of suicides (227), with everyone but Del's mother insisting that a seventeen-year-old victim must have been pregnant: "Otherwise why drown herself, a girl seventeen?" asks Fern (228). In its ruminations on physical outcomes and ailments, this book circles pregnancy as the most decisive incident in a woman's life.

The book tends to examine the reproductive fates of women by presenting them in tandem with their mothers, and the tragic duo of Del's cousin Mary Agnes and her mother, Del's Aunt Moira, represents the primary instance of this pairing. Del says that Mary Agnes, whose problems may not be mentioned (38), "was almost like other people. Except that . . . she had to be with her mother" (38). The girl can't leave her mother's side because, Del's mother explains, "She was deprived of oxygen in the birth canal" (39)—she suffers from cerebral palsy, a condition that Del cruelly mimics (147). Hearing her mother's description of the injury, Del says "The words birth canal made me think of a straight-banked river of blood" (39). This injury occurred because her father held her mother's "legs together on way to the hospital because the doctor had told them she might hemorrhage" (39). This horrific outcome occurs because of the doctor's contextually wrong advice and another man's interference in the birth. While it changes the course of Mary Agnes's life, her mother also seems caught in this moment of reproductive injury. Del explains that "The gloom spreading out from Aunt Moira had a gynecological odour" (39). She describes her aunt as a "sufferer from varicose veins, hemorrhoids, a dropped womb, cysted ovaries, inflammations, discharges, lumps and stones in various places, one of those heavy, cautiously moving, wrecked survivors of the female life, with stories to tell" (39). The trauma of her injurious birth experience has made Aunt Moira a perpetual sufferer from the state of being female.

Mary Agnes's disability also makes her vulnerable to sexual abuse. Del relays how a group of boys lured her to an isolated place then stripped and abandoned her in the cold "and she caught bronchitis and nearly died. That was why, now, she had to wear warm underwear even in summer" (41). This matter-of-fact line of narrative develops from a scene of implied sexual violation to a physical illness, to an outcome that seems merely punishing for Mary Agnes—the hot undergarments in every season. The sequence raises the question of whether Mary Agnes's mother imagines the thick underwear will prevent illness, or rape. This mystifying sequence of causality reflects the traumatic and male-inflicted reasons for her injury during birth, and also leaves a telling gap in justice. The incident leads to

Mary Agnes's warm underwear in every season, but, so far as Del tells it, retribution is not one of the outcomes. The question of whether the boys are held to account is not even opened as a possibility within the story, because, Munro implies, being female in the world of these characters is to be inevitably vulnerable to unpunishable damage by men. Munro characteristically dangles the question of why any of these events followed one from another, while also showing how men injure women with impunity.

Another key mother-daughter pairing along an axis of reproductive health are Naomi and her mother. Best friends, Del and Naomi access a sexual education through the books at their school library, poring over *Kristin Lavransdatter*, and especially "the place where Kristin has her first baby, hour after hour, page after page, blood and agony, squatting on the straw" (112). In response to this scene, and the question of whether Kristin's pregnancy had obliged her to marry, Naomi introduces her mother's expertise: "if a girl has to get married, she either dies having it, or she nearly dies, or else there is something the matter with it. . . . My mother has seen it" (112). A nurse, Naomi's mother is privy to lurid information about pregnancy and birth, "obscene" injuries from coat hangers, and hybrid outcomes of bestiality (112) that both invoke real-world caution and seem to straddle a borderline with myth. She asks Del intrusively about her periods (112) and insists that it's always the girl's fault if she conceives (126). Munro contrasts this crass combination of nosiness and lack of sympathy regarding women's reproductive health with the particular variety of knowledge that Naomi's mother has access to through her job.

Despite her mother's profession, when Naomi herself becomes pregnant and is suffering from its side effects of depression, hormonal volatility, and constipation (219–20), even her abortion attempts, encouraged by her mother, seem to lack grounding in science. "I took quinine," Naomi says. "I took slippery elm and damn laxative and jujubes and I sat in a mustard bath till I thought I was going to turn into a hot dog" (219), a seemingly fantastical remedy that her mother had in fact suggested (219). Though she is a nurse, Naomi's mother's real expertise is not health-related but rather social. Naomi's mother met her father, a much older man, because she "had nursed him before she married him" (146), showing that her profession has also served a social purpose in her own life. "Naomi's mother," Del explains,

> had spies everywhere, old childbed cases, deathbed companions, keeping her informed. In her nursing job, going from one house to another, she was able to operate like an underwater vacuum tube, sucking up what nobody else could get at.
>
> *(137)*

This movement between houses makes her party to everybody's intimate secrets, and, as Del says,

> anybody who will go into birth and death, who will undertake to see and deal with whatever is there—a hemorrhage, the meaty afterbirth, awful dissolution—anybody who does that will have to be listened to, no matter what news they bring.
>
> *(112–13)*

Though her medical advice regarding reproductive health cannot be relied upon, the metaphysical perspective that she gains through attending births, along with the secrets that such experiences reveal to her, make her a source of counsel. Naomi's mother's particular brand of nursing expertise cannot be relied on for practical health guidance but rather gossip.

The most important maternal pairing in the novel is of Del and her mother, whose ruminations on her experiences, on her hopes, and on the other women in her life prove instructive for her daughter. Her own mother "went away for an operation but she had large lumps in both breasts and she died, my mother always said, on the table. On the *operating* table" (73). Her loss of her mother at an early age from cancer in both breasts shows Munro doubling down on female affliction, while her death on the operating table, an outcome presented as horrific by Del's mother, locates her end under the purview of an impersonal and male-dominated medical profession. Del's mother is also preoccupied by the deaths of other women in her life. Her grandmother's sudden death meant that she didn't get the money she'd been promised for her schooling (75), while her most beloved teacher "had married, rather late, and died having a baby. The baby died too and lay in her arm like a wax doll" at the funeral (74). Del's mother ruminates on the prospect of the mortal outcomes of women's hopes for happiness. Reflecting on her mother's ruminations, Del explains that "Stories of the past could go like this, round and round and down to death; I expected it" (75). Del hints that her mother's particular view of sex, and the ominousness she attaches to it, result from her childhood, when her younger brother "tortured" her: "Nothing really accounted for her darkened face at this point in the story, for her way of saying *tortured*. I had not yet learned to recognize the gloom that overcame her in the vicinity of sex" (73). The dark and mortal picture Del's mother associates with sex and reproduction seems partly owing to an unspoken history of sexual abuse by her sibling. Readers may interpret this instance through Munro's own daughter's revelations of her mother's failure to act in response to hearing of her husband's sexual abuse (Skinner). Del's mother, more than any other character, has a clear-eyed as well as emotional view of how, whether from childbearing or abuse, men often cause the torment and affliction of women.

Throughout this novel, Munro links sex and illness. While Naomi leads Del in sexual exploration, saying matter-of-factly that "Everybody does it" (218), it is her illness that permits Del's own first illicit encounter. Mr. Chamberlain has already touched her without permission (150), but Naomi being home sick means Del is alone and available when he invites her on a car ride and asks her to investigate whether Fern has kept any of his love letters (152–53). Naomi is still sick when Mr. Chamberlain picks Del up again (156), this time performing a sexual act in front of her when she doesn't volunteer to participate (159). Del means to relay the story of her sexualized encounters with Mr. Chamberlain to her friend, "But Naomi came out of her illness fifteen pounds lighter, with a whole new outlook on life. . . . She was not even interested in the fact that Mr. Chamberlain had gone, so preoccupied was she with herself and her illness" (162). Naomi's illness creates the space in Del's life for her seamy collaborations with Mr. Chamberlain. It also ensures Del will not reveal her secret, since Naomi loses interest in sex, "although she talked a good deal about Dr. Wallis, and how he had sponged her legs himself, and she had been quite helplessly exposed to him, when she was sick" (162). The hint of sexuality in the description of the doctor is made available by illness and recalls Del's own earlier description of her almost pleasurable discomfort at vaccination appointments: "Every time I thought of the doctor pulling down my pants and jabbing the needle in my buttocks, for small pox, I felt outraged, frantic, unbearably, almost exquisitely humiliated" (41). Illness and medical care permit or force these girls to reveal their bodies to doctors in a humiliation that sometimes seems like enjoyment.

Del also connects sex with illness: "Only when I was sick, with a fever, had I ever before had such a floating feeling, feeling of being languid and protected and at the same time possessing unlimited power" (203). It's worth observing the strangeness of this analogy between sexual pleasure and illness, especially in relation to how Naomi's illness permits Del's experiences with Mr. Chamberlain. Likewise, Del loves the sight of her own blood after having sex for the first time: "When I saw the blood the glory of the whole episode became clear to me" (212). After fighting with Garnet (222–23), she returns to a sense of herself, "though all around it my body clung cracked and bewildered, in the stupid pain of loss" (224). As their friendship fades, Del excuses herself from seeing Naomi after an intense night out because, she says, "I feel too sick" (181). In this book, the ends and beginnings of sickness, romance, and friendship transpire in tandem. Analogizing illness, blood, and the "cracked" body in "pain" to the pleasures and losses of friendship and sex lets Munro explore the stakes of selfhood being superseded by the interests of the body.

Of all the women Munro regards, Fern has lost most: she had a baby, she had Mr. Chamberlain, but she wasn't able to keep either. As with other women, Munro also incorporates her tie to her own mother, acknowledging Fern's absence one day because "she had gone to see her mother in the County Hospital" (83). Characteristically revealing private information acquired from her mother, Naomi is the one who tells Del that Fern "had a baby" (137). But it is Mr. Chamberlain who is most intent on stealing Fern's secrets, and he co-opts Del to his mission, using his sexual engagements with her as a kind of blackmail or inducement to treachery. At his request, Del searches Fern's room for letters, finding newspaper clippings about battles over birth control (156), a woman killing herself when pregnant for the ninth time (155), "about women dying in tenements from complications of pregnancy or childbirth or terrible failed abortions which they performed with hatpins, knitting needles, bubbles of air" (156). Fern, a tragic figure whose life it seems has been marked by an unwanted pregnancy, has kept newspaper clippings about birth control rather than Mr. Chamberlain's love letters.

This notion of birth control is crucial throughout the book, not just to Fern. Del is ridiculed for her mother's public birth control advocacy (165), and she describes how the concept embarrasses her: "All I read now about foam and jelly," she says,

> even the use of the word "vagina" made the whole business seem laborious and domesticated, somehow connected with ointments and bandages and hospitals, and it gave me the same feeling of disgusted, ridiculous helplessness I had when it was necessary to undress at the doctor's.
>
> *(156)*

Although Del is embarrassed by it, the idea of birth control offers the prospect of agency to the women in this world. A bad date, when told that Del supports equal rights for women, retorts, "You believe in capital punishment for women too?" (177). He draws a sinister connection between enforced death and a woman's freedom to choose whether to give birth that reflects the atmosphere of disinterest in women's capacity for self-determination. Overstepping usual boundaries, a boyfriend's mother asks Del if she has a diaphragm and warns her that she "mustn't get into trouble," as she wouldn't let her son marry: "I have seen these cases of young men forced to sacrifice their lives because some girl has got pregnant and I don't think it's right" (188). As usual, the agency and responsibility of men in the negative impacts of reproduction are elided.

When discussing Fern, Del's mother says, "in her grave, hopeful, lecturing voice" (164), that

> There is a change coming I think in the lives of girls and women. Yes. But it is up to us to make it come. All women have had up till now has been their connection with men. All we have had. No more lives of our own, really, than domestic animals.
>
> *(164)*

She goes on to reference Tennyson in describing women like the pets of their husbands (165). Though Del tries to deflect her by telling her birth control is now available, her mother replies that on its own birth control "is not enough" (165), as, she says, "It is self-respect I am really speaking of" (165). Birth control is a start towards women's agency in this book, but it is full self-determination that will mark the key change in the lives of women. Throughout the novel, Munro scrutinizes the ineluctable ailments of reproduction faced by women as their key burden along with the indifference and impact of men.

Margaret Atwood's *The Handmaid's Tale* (1985)

A decade and a half after Munro's ominous suggestion that women's lives have been no more their own "than domestic animals" (164), Margaret Atwood made this comparison of women's fertility to animal husbandry literal in *The Handmaid's Tale* (1985). Atwood's novel represents a dystopian world in which women's bodies are used to reproduce the species. A fascist society seeks to domesticate women as bearers of children, but the domiciles where they live are not homes, and their forced labour (in both senses of the word) position them as having as few rights as farm animals. No more influential book explores the stakes of childbearing, and Atwood's novel persistently questions the status of women, in the household and in society, and in relation to other women, to doctors, and to their own children.

Today, rising struggles with infertility and increasing state efforts to control women's bodies internationally mean the book continues to gather cultural relevance. The wealth of critical responses to this book have been spurred partly by its proliferating film and television adaptations. Fewer critical assessments discuss its depictions of sex and birth, despite their prominence in the book itself. Ana-Karina Schneider shows how the novel participates alongside other works of feminist dystopian fiction in questioning the meaning of women's bodies and reproduction. Pamela Cooper uses the work of Michel Foucault to analyze "sexual surveillance" in Atwood's portrayal of physicians in the novel.

Just as in Laurence's "To Set Our House in Order," the position of the childbearing woman within the home here is a source of meaning. The Commander's wife blocks the handmaid Offred's entrance to the house when she arrives, because "She wanted me to feel that I could not come into the house unless she said so" (15). Control over the access points to the house implies dominion over its internal space, but also a position of maternity in relation to those born there. The uncertain status of the handmaids means that no one knows whether they should enter through the front or back doors (14): battles over status play out in the territory of the house. The position of the driver, Nick, is reflected in how he lives with the family, "in the household, over the garage," but not in the house itself and "hasn't been issued a woman, not even one" (20). His inside-outside position in the house indicates his lower status, just as the handmaid's status throws her relation to the house into question.

The weird placement in the house of the handmaids is reflected in their comparison to animals, since livestock too live within the possession of a household, but not in the house. The aunts patrol with "electric cattle prods" (4), while in the bathroom during her strange night out, Offred sees a woman she knows must be an aunt because "The cattle prod's on the table, its thong around her wrist" (279). The women are positioned as animals by the instruments of pain that are used against them, while Offred describes the tattoo on her ankle as "a cattle-brand. It means ownership" (294). Classing the women as farm animals is a comment on their labour. "Think of it as being in the army" (8), an Aunt says, while Cora suggests that "It's not what you'd call hard work" (11), and the Commander's wife describes their relation as "a business transaction" (17). There is a potent ambiguity around what kind of work the handmaids are doing, whether their status is equivalent to farm animals, or not. It is the fact of being used so completely for her physical capacity that permits these comparisons to farm animals, and Offred avoids looking at her body in the bath because "I don't want to look at something that determines me so completely" (71). Whether a participant in a business transaction or a domesticated creature, Offred's body and its potential for fertility, rather than her mind or identity, determine her position in this society.

In this world where women's physical states are their entire being, illness offers something to talk about, and drugs both enforce participation and promise escape. Offred imagines being able to sit in the kitchen with Rita and Cora to

> talk, about aches and pains, illnesses, our feet, our backs, all the different kinds of mischief that our bodies, like unruly children, can get up to. . . . We would exchange remedies and try to outdo each other in the recital of our physical miseries.
>
> *(11)*

Cures and medical complaints are the substrate of talk between women. Women need extra rest in the Red Centre possibly because "We were on some kind of pill or drug I think, they put it in the food, to keep us calm" (81). Even laughing would put Offred at risk of being diagnosed with hysteria: "And then a needle, a pill. It could be fatal" (169). Drugs let the regime keep women in line, but they also portend escape. Offred gave her daughter a pill to make her drowsy during their flight attempt (85), while Moira suggests trying to escape by faking an illness: "They send an ambulance, I've seen it" (102). In this toxic world, contagion is a constant risk, but one that is as frequently social as physical. "She thinks I may be catching, like a disease or any form of bad luck" (10), Offred writes of a housekeeper, while her friend Moira says of another handmaid's distress, "You can't let her go slipping over the edge. That stuff is catching" (251). Speaking of Offred's husband Luke, Moira compares dating men to catching syphilis, and Offred asks her, "Are you calling Luke a social disease?" (199). At the "Prayvaganza," there are roped areas to keep the handmaids from contaminating others (247). During sex with the Commander, Offred muses, "Maybe I'm crazy and this is some new kind of therapy" (107), and she wishes she could just get well. The brutality of this new system has no room for remedies, however: as Moira warns, if women lose their grip on reality, "They won't mess around with trying to cure you," they'll just shoot to kill (250). Illness, contagion, pills, and absent cures define this world where women's physical production is the greatest goal, and losing track of reality through drugs or despair promises death more than escape.

With women coerced into producing babies, the prospect of abortion is no longer an option, but rather a historical memory and a cautionary tale from the present. Offred remembers her mother participating in marches to advocate for abortion after clinic bombings (208), and Moira had worked for a women's publisher that "put out books on birth control and rape and things like that" (205). But now, Offred writes, "No woman in her right mind, these days, would seek to prevent a birth, should she be so lucky as to conceive" (38). Still, the prospect of pregnancy without surviving infants lurks through Offred's world. She passes a funeral for a foetus in jar (48) and eavesdrops on Rita and Cora's gossip as they mutter about failed pregnancies: "*Stillborn, it was.* Or, *Stabbed her with a knitting needle, right in the belly*" (12). While pregnancies that don't end in live births take on the status of dark rumours, in a public ceremony Janine confesses to having had an abortion after being gang raped at fourteen, and the crowd of women are led in a chant insisting that it was all her fault (82). The executed bodies Offred walks by often seem to have been doctors who once provided abortions. "The men wear white coats, like those worn by doctors or scientists," she writes, "each has a placard hung around his neck to show why he has been executed: a drawing of a human foetus. They were doctors, then, in the time before, when such things were legal" (37).

The shift in legality of abortion has had implications for medical professionals that reflect current arguments in the United States regarding not only the status of abortion, but also other reproductive technologies such as in vitro fertilization (IVF). At the time of writing, doctors in Alabama risk prosecution for murder for inadvertently dropping a test tube of embryos (Rabin and Ghorayshi). "It's no excuse," writes Offred regarding the executed doctors she passes, "that what they did was legal at the time: their crimes are retroactive. They have committed atrocities" (37). The question of what constitutes atrocity in the context of reproduction is one that this book keeps posing, and one that is gathering renewed relevance today. Offred explains that the doctors' prior abortion work would have been discovered through hospital records

> or—more likely, since most hospitals destroyed such records once it became clear what was going to happen—by informants: ex-nurses perhaps, or a pair of them, since evidence from a single woman is no longer admissible.
>
> *(37)*

Women's voices need to be doubled to be accepted as evidence, but only if they provide information that supports the regime's perspective, while the status of nurses as medical professionals gives them access to private information and lets them operate as enforcers of the state.

Nurses represent women whose authority may be co-opted by government officials, but Atwood also examines the relative status of women in other positions of influence. The Historical Notes section explains that, in Gilead, people who had handmaids' services "could lay claim to them through their position in the elite" (349), just as infertility treatments now are also often the sole purview of the rich. Illustrating another category of status for women, Offred explains that the wives who haven't conceived are the ones to "watch out for" because they are "defeated women" (51). In a scene that reflects tense sessions in fertility clinics today, the women in the doctor's waiting room assess their place in the group: "Covertly we regard each other, sizing up each other's bellies: is anyone lucky?" (66). Offred watches for blood each month, "fearfully, for when it comes it means failure" because "the expectations of others," she says, "have become my own" (84). Pregnancy improves the status of women in Gilead, while simply not conceiving indicates a woman's personal failure, an obstructed status, which, Atwood implies, may be extrapolated to the pressures on real women to reproduce. Observing a pregnant handmaid, Offred explains that "She's a magic presence to us, an object of envy and desire, we covet her. She's a flag on a hilltop, showing us what can still be done: we too can be saved" (29). This pregnant woman is called a "Show-off" (30) for risking an outing, because, "Now that she's the carrier of life, she is closer to death, and needs special security" (30). While pregnant women receive an extremely elevated status, Moira explains that women who cannot conceive are sent to the "Colonies" (288), a banishment reminiscent of England's historic expulsion of convicted people to Australia and other colonies (see Foxhall; Rushton and Morgan). The irony from the standpoint of colonial logic is that, historically, populating colonies with new births was the goal, but with the low fertility rates in Gilead, this expectation has been reversed. Throughout this book, the status of women depends on their fertility.

Just as reproduction throws into question the status of women, doctors in this world also occupy a privileged but contentious position. Their prior roles have been usurped, while the Marthas' green dresses are "like a surgeon's gown of the time before" (10). When Offred sees a doctor every month for tests (66), the sheets covering her mean he "deals with a torso only" (67), and he "isn't supposed to speak to me except when it's absolutely necessary. But this doctor is talkative" (67). The chattiness of this physician signals his transgression of other rules, too, and he offers to try to impregnate Offred (68), warning her that "You don't have a lot of time left" (69). The doctor's threat carries the risk that "He could fake the tests, report me for cancer, for infertility, have me shipped off to the Colonies, with the Unwomen" (69). This is the extent of the doctor's power, to try to coerce illicit sex with the threat of exerting what sway he has with the regime, to have a worse outcome inflicted on Offred. Despite this attempt at coercion, the power of doctors is severely curtailed in this society compared to their prior roles. False diagnosis here becomes a form of attack, but in this new regime, where the status of doctors has changed, that is the full extent of his power.

What permits this encounter though is the medicalization of fertility in the context of the society's low birth rates. After conception, however, diagnostic help from doctors is spurned. Offred explains that there is constant uncertainty about whether newborns will be healthy: "They could tell once, with machines, but that is now outlawed. What would be the point of knowing, anyway? You can't have them taken out" (129). Doctors have lost their position as attendants to pregnancy and birth and can only conduct tests—and issue threats—in the absence of conception. To condemn past medical practices, the women at the Centre are shown a film of "a pregnant woman, wired up to a machine, electrodes coming out of her every which way so that she looked like a broken robot, an intravenous drip feeding into her arm" (131). Though doctors "used to be in charge" at births (131), now they are only allowed to attend deliveries "if it can't be helped" and anaesthesia for labour is avoided because the Bible declares that "*in sorrow thou shalt bring forth children*" (131). Both diminished and increased in status in this new world, doctors are not allowed to attend births or administer anaesthetic, but are expected to assess women's bodies, and can break the law by having opportunities to try to impregnate the women, or by retaliating with false diagnoses and unnecessary medication. Just as it does for women, this book chronicles the altered status of doctors.

Throughout, Atwood calls into question not only the position of science in Gilead, but also the causes for the infertility epidemic. The women are obliged to eat bland meals, because "Studies have been done" (74), while alcohol, coffee, and smoking are also prohibited (16). Precise reasons for the low birth rates are attributed to widespread chemicals, and while at the Red Centre the women are told that their "very flesh may be polluted, dirty as an oily beach, sure death to shore birds and unborn babies" (129). They are shown a chart of the years-long birth-rate decline (130) but are taught that "There was no one cause" (129). Scientific measurement can track but not explain. The final "Historical Notes" section documents more attempts to explain the infertility of Gilead (349). Reflecting on the efforts to control birth rates in the secular society before the evangelical takeover, Professor Pieixoto suggests that "Some infertility, then, was willed . . . but the rest was not" (349). Other proposed causes include a fictional strain of syphilis (349), AIDS and nuclear plants (350), the development of biological weapons resulting in a "sterility-causing virus" (355), "gene-splicing experiments with mumps" (355), and insecticides (350), which dominated the public imagination after the 1962 publication of Rachel Carson's *Silent Spring*.

The suspicion that science itself could have caused the fertility disaster holds an interesting parallel with misinformation denigrating COVID-19 vaccines, as well as theories regarding the lab-based origin of the virus (see Butter and Knight). Atwood's litany of hypothetical pathogens reflects contemporaneous concerns about environmental and social ills, at a time when green activism had not yet consolidated its efforts around the notion of global warming. Professor Pieixoto suggests that the rise of fertility treatments preceded the turn to Gilead's handmaids (350), but that the society outlawed what we now call IVF "as irreligious, but legitimized and enforced" the use of surrogacy, "which was considered to have biblical precedents" (350). Part of what the book documents is a turn from scientific sources of authority to religious ones, in a context where science and doctors are called upon when they can be seen to support religious and patriarchal objectives, and cast aside, even executed, if not.

Ultimately fiction and science share in the hunt for causes. One reason Atwood's novel has such lasting power is that its hypothesis about the future continues to feel astute, even as the technological orientation of the society it portrays is in fact nostalgic, not innovative: IVF has been thrown out in favour of biblical surrogacy. Science fiction is normally thought to fantasize about advancement, but the biggest change in Atwood's society is social and retrogressive. The eye-opening display of a fearful future is not in the representation of technology in this book, but in its depiction of social attitudes towards reproductive rights and fights over the status of women and their bodies that feel gravely relevant today.

Ami McKay's *The Birth House* (2006) and Lawrence Hill's *The Book of Negroes* (2007)

Two influential twenty-first century historical novels published within six months of each other both regard maternal health, each with a focus on Nova Scotia. Ami McKay's bestseller *The Birth House* (2006) explores the maritime history of rural midwifery, while Lawrence Hill's *The Book of Negroes* (2007) follows an enslaved midwife whose skills take her around the world.

The primary conflict of Ami McKay's *The Birth House* (2006) is between midwives and representatives of the medical profession, with the new maternity home, a birth facility, localizing the perceived ills of organized medical care. McKay regards this conflict through a somewhat polemical lens that invites readings of this work for its reflection of contemporary rather than historical arguments. As signalled by its title, the novel concerns the location of birth, with the main characters arguing for the benefit of home deliveries.

The Birth House critiques the paternalist medical establishment seeking to impose its methods on the women of the Scots Bay, the rural Nova Scotia community McKay depicts. The new maternity home, where women are to give birth attended by doctors (29), is supposed to relieve them of having "their babies in fishing shacks and barns" (34). Although the midwife Miss B says there "Ain't no *exact* way to have a baby" (92), the doctor suggests that those who seek the care of midwives will commit the "crime" of not getting proper birth assistance (134). He gives a presentation about "the advantages of modern childbirth" (56) and drugs that "put the labour process in the doctor's hands" so that "He has complete control" (57). This off-putting depiction negates the agency of the women who are giving birth and those trained to help them. The doctors and midwives are also divided by their answers to whether pain is an acceptable aspect of birth: "isn't there always pain in childbirth?" (132) a postpartum mother asks the doctor. McKay links the doctor's goal of reducing the pain of childbirth to the harm of depriving a mother of a memory of birth (133). The last pages of the book are devoted to a list of home remedies, a celebratory paean to traditional cures (369–80), in contrast to the mass-produced drugs of organized medicine. The primary tension of this book comes from the ongoing fight between two competing frameworks of maternity care.

In McKay's telling, the role of the midwife can span deliveries, general healthcare, and advocacy. So broad and significant are the midwife's skills that Dora leaves her community to tend to those suffering in the aftermath of the Halifax Explosion (213–15). She also goes to Boston (296), and once more demonstrates her broad medical knowledge and ability during the influenza epidemic (326–27). The story closes with a news item about her speech at a rally in support of midwives (361–62). Midwives also have preferences for how birth should happen. Their form of propriety requires that women should be able to give birth in a real home, either their own, or that of the midwife attending them. As she inherits the role of sole midwife to the community, Dora explains that "[her] house became the birth house. That's what the women came to call it" (ix). In McKay's final, almost cartoonish exposition of the conflict between midwives and doctors, during a delivery the physician pounds on the door of Dora's house (345), at the ready with unwelcome emblems of medicalized childbirth, forceps and the labour drug pituitrin (346). The ongoing argument over the proper places and ways to give birth gives way to a literal fight at the threshold of the birth house, as Dora "grabbed the frame of the door and held tight, refusing him entry" (346). The proof that the midwives have prevailed comes when the maternity home closes (363) and the women are told they may seek medical care "in Halifax" (363). McKay puts the doctor's "Maternity Home" in conflict with the midwives' "Birth House." Though they have similar names, the two spaces represent the competing approaches to healthcare for women that this book chronicles.

More than most works that concern maternity, McKay's story puts the real risks and complications of fertility, pregnancy, and childbirth on display. One woman asks the midwives for a remedy to ensure regular periods, with the tacit understanding that the prescribed tincture will induce an abortion (99–101). Another woman experiences postpartum depression (222), and a thirteen-year-old in labour starts to haemorrhage (256). When Ginny suffers from headaches, the doctor doesn't notice (335), although Dora knew "as soon as [she] saw her that Ginny was well on her way to trouble" (340) after the doctor's ineffectual ministrations (319–20). With Dora's help Ginny's baby arrives safely (343–45). Dora and Miss B don't need to know the Latin name for preeclampsia—which they refer to as "Stranger's Face" (341)—to understand what's happening and how to respond, even though they can't always save their patients. So complete is McKay's interest in women's reproductive health that the novel devotes a significant interlude to Dora's experimentation with an early vibrator (200–2). Though the doctor introduces her to the machine and gives her an initial "treatment" (195–98), he later tries to blackmail her by threatening to share his knowledge of her enjoyment of it (232–34). This book pursues a variegated and clinical level of detail regarding women's bodies, their ailments, and pleasures.

In McKay's novel, midwifery reflects a kind of folkloric expertise that is as often mystical as precise. McKay puts the strangeness of delivery into conversation with the supernatural, describing the "Moon's voice" that "pulled their babies into the light of birth" (ix). The mystery of Miss B's abilities puts her off-limits, and most in the community don't associate with her "unless you're a woman who's expecting, or you've got an ailment that can't be cured" (24). Miss B, whose great grandfather was also a "traiteur" or healer (25–26), is cast as teaching or practising "witchery" (70, 96), but her own understanding of her gifts is pious: she had a vision of Saint Brigit asking her to "dedicate her hands to bringing forth the children of this place" (26). Dora's husband questions her impact (171), and he doesn't want his wife to work as a midwife (154). Though they seek cures, a "Midwife curse" (252) attends both Dora and Miss B, and Dora is blamed for the birth of "three-legged albino calf" (5, 291). Dora says she wants to be a mother (154), but she becomes one only through adoption (263–64), as though attending so many births had somehow lessened her own reproductive capacity. Her wedding dress is made of christening gowns (159), a symbolic presaging of births that do not come to pass. McKay lets Dora's infertility seem a product of her special powers and does not problematize it as an illness that could be cured.

An atmosphere of the supernatural encircles the midwives, while in contrast Dr. Thomas represents the potential harms of an overconfident and paternalistic medical profession that insists on payment. He suggests that under medical care "women can rely on more than faith to see them through the grave dangers of childbirth" (32). He thereby casts midwifery as mysticism and presents the conflict between their forms of knowledge as a battle between "superstition" and "science" (88–89). Under the care of midwives, the doctor insists, "children are being neglected in the womb" (128). He touts "modern alternatives" to "trials of childbirth" (129) and claims to be offering "a recipe for healthy babies and happy homes" (130). He suggests that doctors "leave nothing to chance" due to their training (131), and that midwifery is a "tiresome responsibility" (132). Belying his confidence in his own medical knowledge, when he invades Dora's house, he noses through her remedies (293). The doctor in his first appearance suggests that "The suffering that women have endured in childbirth can be a thing of the past" (29), prompting the midwife Miss B to accuse him of selling something (29). His overconfidence is what makes the doctor seem mercantile.

Indeed, the question of what the doctor is selling, whether payment should ever be received in exchange for care, is another point of conflict between the midwives and the doctors. The doctor advises women to "seek out the best care you can afford" (129); his help through the medical insurance company runs to twenty-five dollars per woman per year, which he acknowledges may exceed what most can afford, so he suggests that women should help pay for each other (59). Even beyond questions of affordability, the expectations created by paying the doctor cause problems: for example, when he arrives too late for a birth (161), the new father can't believe he won't provide further care, because "We already paid" (162). In contrast Miss B refuses all payment for her midwifery (30), including when she provides an abortion (100), and this tenet is repeated in Dora's birth house, where "No payment shall be required" (363). This commitment reflects Canadian ideals regarding access to healthcare that suggest the system be funded by the collective so that individuals need not pay up front in times of need.

Despite McKay's attention to realistic complications of early twentieth-century pregnancy, what this book brushes over in rejecting professionalized medicine is the contemporaneous emergence of caesarean section as a standard delivery method. The paternalism of a medical profession that excluded women practitioners certainly led to negative outcomes for maternity patients, but the complicating features of this history should be kept in mind when reading this book. During the first two decades of the twentieth century, which McKay's book narrates, the procedure of caesarean section started regularly saving lives in Canada, including in small Nova Scotia towns, due to greater understanding of the technique and improved antiseptic methods (Baskett S248). Although this still-risky delivery method was rare, likely limited to male practitioners, and often hospital-based for their antiseptic environments, it did save the lives of women and babies who would otherwise have died.

Another essential historical context for this novel concerns the Ideal Maternity Home in East Chester, Nova Scotia, which the midwife Lila Young and her husband operated from 1928 to 1947. As the journalist Bette L. Cahill documents in *Butterbox Babies: Baby Sales, Baby Deaths* (published in 1992 and revised in 2006), the Youngs trafficked infants for paid adoptions against the will and without the knowledge of birth parents and prevented mothers from receiving antibiotic and other lifesaving treatments from doctors. Many women died as a result, and hundreds of babies succumbed to the Youngs' purposeful neglect and were buried in grocery boxes in unmarked graves in the vicinity of the home. Cahill suggests that the greater oversight of hospital facilities along with the use of standard medical procedures could have avoided these outcomes (30–33). Though by no means representative of midwifery in general, the criminal activity of this home devastated countless Nova Scotia families and must be remembered as part of the history of maternal health in the province.

These complicating historical contexts should be kept in mind when reading McKay's book. McKay strives for authenticity, for example by basing her tale in the actual hamlet of Scots Bay, but her discounting of real achievements in obstetrical medical care negates an important history and a key aspect of the tension that she portrays. Recent scholarship on this novel tends to adopt its oppositional stance toward obstetrical practice (see Hashish; Mohan and Karmakar). The contemporary challenge between obstetrics and midwifery however often lies in bringing about more effective collaborations between the two approaches (Warmelink et al.), rather than in the forcefully competing claims of legitimacy presented here.

Published fewer than six months after Ami McKay's *The Birth House*, Lawrence Hill's *The Book of Negroes* also offers a historical perspective on midwifery, including in Nova Scotia, but one that chronicles a time roughly two hundred years earlier, when slavery was still practised in America and was being slowly abolished in British colonies.

Hill gives his main character, Aminata, midwifery skills that bring her connections throughout many communities and eventually around the world. She learned the craft from her mother in West Africa (14–15) and can tell when a woman is pregnant (30). As a child she's calm at births (86) and can diagnose twins in utero (139), she knows when birth will happen (47), and is reputed for her skill (60). On the slave ship to America, she is enjoined to work with the doctor onboard (63) and is taken under the wing of an enslaved midwife named Georgia once she lands (143–44). Just as Dorie knows more cures than those for childbed illnesses alone, Georgia inoculates Aminata against smallpox using a folk technique (145). Throughout Aminata's tale, Hill refers to the work of the midwife as "catching" babies (15, 144, 206, 283, 325, etc). The slave owner Solomon Lindo hires her out as midwife (204), and, after helping to deliver the out-of-wedlock baby of an officer (274–77), she starts working to secure care and homes for sex workers and their babies (277). She provides delivery and abortion care (280) but once free she takes an opportunity to move to Nova Scotia from Boston partly because she "was tired of making life easier for British officers by catching the babies of their mistresses" (283). In Nova Scotia she still attends deliveries though she is no longer paid (334). But after losing her own child to kidnapping she doesn't attend any deliveries for a year (350–51), despite the urgency of women's needs and the paucity of care in this eighteenth-century maritime setting. Aminata's education and connection with her community mean she can help register those who wish to travel to Nova Scotia in the "The Book of Negroes" (287) that titles the book. As a result of her clerical and medical services (392–93), her participation in colonial administration transpires both through ushering illegitimate offspring into the world, and in inscribing names into the administrative record.

Common complications of childbirth are notably missing from this fictional account. Death in childbirth and stillbirth are not part of this narrative, although they were frequent in this period (Loudon). Reading McKay's and Hill's novels about midwives together, therefore, both illuminates past Canadian contexts of midwifery and birth, and shows how novels can overwrite historical suffering. Aminata's long desire to be a storyteller (447), however, and her eventual work to write her own story (457) puts this character among other storytelling practitioners in the history of Canadian literature, such as Vincent Lam's Chen and Shani Mootoo's Tyler.

Sheila Heti's *Motherhood* (2018)

Sheila Heti's *Motherhood* (2018) examines the stakes of choosing whether to reproduce for women's bodies, friendships, and identities. The novel is among the most accessible and discussed of the avant-garde author's books, sparking several scholarly studies of its interventions in relation to, for example, psychoanalysis (Shirm), queer time (Frankel), and uncertainty (Currie). While Lawrence Hill's fictional odyssey explores the agency and geographic trajectory of an enslaved woman, Heti's ruminating narrative relays a mental journey to find out what a woman should do with the freedom to have children, and whether children bear responsibility for the anguish of their mothers.

"No child, through her own will, can pull a mother out of her suffering" (15), Heti writes, and her book grapples with the feelings that result from her character's knowledge that she wasn't the most important part of her own mother's life (257). Heti's book is divided into repeating biological stages of the reproductive cycle, a tortuous questioning structured by the body's rhythms, which are as circular and repetitive as the character's thought processes: PMS, Bleeding, Follicular, Ovulating, PMS. This structural concern with the reproductive cycle is reflected in the character's suggestion that "This book is a prophylactic" (193). Like the rhythm method that times sex to a woman's cycle to avoid pregnancy, the circular questioning is meant as a contraception technique with a high enough fail rate to permit chance to make the ultimate decision.

The character is desperate to find an answer to a mysterious question. "Whether I want kids," she writes, "is a secret I keep from myself—it is the greatest secret I keep from myself" (21). While knowing whether or not one wants children feels like a preference that one keeps from oneself to this character, it also seems to be one that confers the benefit of an elevated status. "Do I want children," the character asks,

> because I want to be admired as the admirable sort of woman who has children? Because I want to be seen as a normal sort of woman . . . a body that can make babies, and someone who another person wants to make babies with?
>
> *(22)*

Having a child, this character hypothesizes, could improve her position in the eyes of others, by making her seem desirable, physically healthy, and above all, "normal." She suggests that a refusal to have children could be in response to the Holocaust (162) and considers whether "motherhood means honoring one's mother" (200), while being a child may entail taking on mother's sorrow (144). Expressing her struggles with her mother, the character writes, "I can't be any better than her, and she can't be any better than me. And this upsets us most of all" (239). Because pregnancy is a choice for this character, it has meaning that she finds impossible to extricate from her relationship with her own mother.

This decision is often determined by biology, and this book puts forward a dualistic notion of mind and body, where both have a will and agency of their own. The character suggests the two are separate, and that "those doing spiritual work should not have to be chasing children around" (36) but that having had a baby she might feel "Genetic relief—relief at having procreated" (23). For this character, children reveal the separation between mental and biological work. She feels that "people who want to forbid abortions" just "want that woman to be doing the work of child-rearing more than they want her to be doing anything else" (32). For Heti, the biological nature of reproduction distinguishes it from intellectual labour. Womanhood itself seems to depend on a relationship to motherhood: "What is a woman—who is not a mother—doing that is more important than mothering?" (134). The character also imagines that there might be some innate instinctual propulsion operating in her decision-making, one that is profoundly contrary to her intellectual motivations. She questions whether one is a woman first or an individual (25), becomes tongue tied while discussing birth control with a female doctor (28), wonders about the meaning of a woman's life without motherhood (159), and suggests that not wanting children would represent a "biologically different" orientation (161). Deeply ambivalent about undergoing what she describes as the "transformation" of pregnancy (147), the character visits a fertility clinic (127), wryly observing that "Getting my eggs frozen would have been like freezing my indecision" (128).

Even as the menstrual cycle structures the book, the character's periods impact her life. Her partner "insists we only fight like this before my period" (213), and the character observes that "Now my periods are getting irregular" (194). This lapsing of her fertility is welcome, and, she says, "I experience biology's forgetting about me as an immense relief, as a sort of bliss. If you do not have a child, at a certain age you become your own child" (267). Becoming one's own child is a welcome outcome of choosing not to have children. The character concludes that "My body has always experienced the idea of having a child as an absurdity and an abomination" (269), raising the question of why the narrative has been put forward in answer to a question that didn't need answering.

Along with the duality Heti proposes between mind and body, the prospect of using medication to alleviate suffering is set against mental distress and the anguished relation between mothers and their children. The character describes how her ruminations are a practice of "Causing myself pain in advance of any real pain" (37). Fear attends this character's indecision and suffering, and she asks whether "this book, all along," has "just been evidence of my deep fear of everything" (244). She writes, "I understand that fear beckons to a person as much as possibility does, and even more strongly" (264). The possibility of a baby is the counterpart to the pervasive fear that causes her greatest distress. She realizes that the answer to her question about whether or not to have children would have been clarified "If I had asked myself that question, thinking about my deathbed, I really would have known. I should have looked at my deathbed, not at the maternity ward" (269). She realizes that her mental health is impacted by her menstrual cycle (230) and reflects on the benefits of medication to alleviate mental distress, writing that "Some women are politically against drugs—but not, it seems, the ones who are suffering" (230). Once medicated, the character marvels at the impact of antidepressants (240–3) and says that before "Everything had always stung me too painfully" (241). "Before the drugs," she says, "sadness and anxiety was all I knew" (241). The pain, sadness, and anxiety that underpin her ruminations over whether to have a child, and which are exacerbated by hormonal cycles of own fertility, are alleviated by the biological intervention, not of pregnancy, but of medication. The revelation that her mother took antidepressants for years (256) caps the character's struggles with her feelings about their relationship. Heti's exploration of mental anguish over reproduction and its relief through medication asks which medical interventions women really need, fertility treatments—or antidepressants.

In Heti's simultaneous exploration of depression and fertility ambivalence, babies and ideas become competing potential occupants of the space of a woman's body. All this thinking leads the character to the idea that "The main thing about motherhood is letting another creature come through you" (43). The stakes of this formulation become more clear as the book closes, and the character visits her mother's new house: "In the study, she opened a door that I thought would lead into another room, but I was startled to see the door open onto the vast and cavernous barn that her house had been built up from" (252). This revelation of this space for creatures to come through seems to the character "like she was showing me her unconscious, the basement of her mind" (252). Just as in Munro's suggestion that women have had "no more lives of our own, really, than domestic animals" (164), here the biological productivity of women analogizes them to barns, spaces for creatures to come through—whether babies or ideas. In Heti's dualistic vision of the mind and body, her character's ruminations above all concern whether she wants to be inhabited by babies or ideas, as though these were mutually exclusive entities that travel through women.

Conclusion

Forcing women to seek help from caregivers and hunt for answers, in these books illnesses and suffering derive from fertility and its failures. Whereas the earliest novel under discussion charts narrative disruptions that result from stillbirth and death in childbirth, the last portrays fertility clinics as the scene of a dubious medicalization of conception itself. The span of these works shows advancements in maternal healthcare, the stakes of access to birth control and midwifery or obstetrical care, and changing notions of what constitutes reproductive illness and trouble.

Heti's book in particular should be read through the context of how, for many women in twenty-first century Canada, getting pregnant is a matter of medical intervention. Whereas more unplanned pregnancies may have occurred in earlier generations, lower fertility rates and more reliable methods of contraception (Statistics Canada) mean that having children is now usually a decision, but one that women may come to only once their fertility starts to fail, and with which they sometimes find themselves seeking medical help. Whereas McKay's novel captures twentieth-century objections to the medicalization of birth, now conception is also medicalized in fertility "clinics," a word for spaces that offer treatment for illness. In the space of the fertility clinic, the illness being treated is the lack of a child in the present, and sometimes also the anxious desire to preserve the opportunity to want a child in a future that may never arrive. Conversations today are increasing about how widespread fertility "treatments" sometimes bring more pain than relief. For example, *The Retrievals* podcast from 2023 (Burton et al.) considers how the medicalization of fertility permits new forms of misery, and Charlene Carr's *Hold My Girl* (2023) imagines the fallout when two women realize their eggs have been switched. Whether salvation or punishment, the fertility clinic today represents a laborious borderland of women's effort and time that is neither work, nor leisure, a place of suffering in the pursuit of a seemingly desired outcome about which many, like Heti's character, nevertheless feel ambivalent.

Desired, feared, or regretted, pregnancy in these works represents a disruption in the lives of women that, like an illness, directs their narratives of suffering. Heti's focus on houses in relation to pregnancy reflects the concerns of other works in this chapter, including *As For Me and My House,* "To Set our House in Order," and *The Birth House*. Even in *The Handmaid's Tale*, Offred's confinement in the home is made strange through the twisted lines of authority in the house, where the fertile woman is not the one in charge. These books help us consider the meaning of the house and the fertility clinic as frames for pregnant women, showcasing the troubles and illnesses of reproduction, and featuring women's agency as often as its theft.

Works Cited

Atwood, Margaret. *The Handmaid's Tale*. 1985. McClelland & Stewart, 2019.

Barthes, Roland. "The Death of the Author." *Image Music Text*. 1968, translated by Stephen Heath, Fontana, 1977, pp. 142–49.

Baskett, Thomas F. "Evolution of Operative Obstetric Delivery in Canada." *Journal of Obstetrics and Gynaecology Canada*, vol. 41, Supplement 2, Dec. 2019, pp. S244–50.

Burton, Susan, et al. "From Serial Productions: The Retrievals." *The New York Times*, 22 June 2023.

Butter, Michael, and Peter Knight, editors. *Covid Conspiracy Theories in Global Perspective*. Routledge, 2023.

Cahill, Bette L. *Butterbox Babies: Baby Sales, Baby Deaths: New Revelations 15 Years Later*. 1992. 2nd ed., Fernwood, 2006.

Cameron, Ian A. "The Family Physician as Fifth Business." *Canadian Family Physician*, vol. 63, no. 11, Nov. 2017, pp. 870–71.

Cameron, Ian A. "Observations from Fifth Business." *Canadian Family Physician*, vol. 35, May 1989, pp. 1029, 1067–68.

Carr, Charlene. *Hold My Girl*. HarperCollins, 2023.

Coldwell, Joan. "Memory Organized: The Novels of Audrey Thomas." *Canadian Literature*, no. 92, 1982, pp. 46–56.

Cooper, Pamela. "Sexual Surveillance and Medical Authority in Two Versions of *the Handmaid's Tale*." *Journal of Popular Culture*, vol. 28, no. 4, Mar. 1995, pp. 49–66.

Currie, Mark. "Maybe Baby: Uncertainty and Decision in Sheila Heti's *Motherhood*." *Textual Practice*, vol. 36, no. 1, Jan. 2022, pp. 116–34.

Davies, Robertson. *Fifth Business*. 1970. Penguin, 1996.

Dean, Michelle. "Alice Munro Was Hiding in Plain Sight." *The Cut*, 8 July 2024.
Demers, Patricia. *Women's Writing in Canada*. U of Toronto P, 2019.
Donne, John. "Death Be Not Proud." *The Variorum Edition of the Poetry of John Donne: The Holy Sonnets*, edited by Gary A. Stringer and Paul A. Parrish, vol. 7.1, Indiana UP, 2005, p. 107.
Duffin, Jacalyn. *Lovers and Livers: Disease Concepts in History*. U of Toronto P, 2005.
Estok, Simon C. "An Ecocritical Reading, Slightly Queer, of *As for Me and My House*." *Journal of Canadian Studies*, vol. 44, no. 3, Aug. 2010, pp. 75–95.
Firefly Books. *Love You Forever, by Robert Munsch*, www.fireflybooks.com/BookDetails?Pid=374. Accessed 29 July 2024.
Foucault, Michel. "What Is an Author?" *Language, Counter-Memory, Practice*. 1969, edited by Donald F. Bouchard, Cornell UP, 1977, pp. 113–39.
Foxhall, Katherine. "From Convicts to Colonists: The Health of Prisoners and the Voyage to Australia, 1823–53." *The Journal of Imperial and Commonwealth History*, vol. 39, no. 1, 2011, pp. 1–19.
Frankel, Alexandra Vieux. "Queering Reproductive Time: Jacob's Wrestling and Queer Temporalities in Sheila Heti's *Motherhood*." *Canadian Jewish Studies*, vol. 35, May 2023, pp. 65–83.
Goldman, Marlene. "Madness, Masculinity, and Magic in Robertson Davies' *Fifth Business*: A Tale of Hysteria; Or, 'the Suffocation of the Mother'." *University of Toronto Quarterly*, vol. 78, no. 4, Oct. 2009, pp. 991–99.
Hashish, Nadia. "Towards Holistic Medical Humanities." *Alif: Journal of Comparative Poetics*, no. 40, 2020, pp. 164–85.
Heti, Sheila. *Motherhood*. Knopf, 2018.
Hill, Colin. "As for Sinclair Ross (Review)." *University of Toronto Quarterly*, vol. 76, no. 1, 2007, pp. 568–69.
Hill, Lawrence. *The Book of Negroes*. HarperCollins, 2007.
Jestrovic, Silvija. *Performances of Authorial Presence and Absence*. Palgrave Macmillan, 2020.
Laurence, Margaret. "To Set Our House in Order." *A Bird in the House*. 1963, McClelland & Stewart, 1974, pp. 39–60.
Lederman, Marsha. "The Misogynists Trying to Turn the United States into Gilead." *The Globe and Mail*, 1 Aug. 2024.
Lesk, Andrew. "On Sinclair Ross's Straight(ened) House." *ESC English Studies in Canada*, vol. 28, no. 1, 2002, pp. 65–90.
Loudon, I. "Deaths in Childbed from the Eighteenth Century to 1935." *Medical History*, vol. 30, no. 1, Jan. 1986, pp. 1–41.
McKay, Ami. *The Birth House*. Knopf, 2006.
Mohan, Swathi, and Manali Karmakar. "Obstetric Violence, Birth Trauma, Agency, and Care in Ami McKay's *The Birth House*." *Cogent Arts & Humanities*, vol. 10, no. 1, Dec. 2023, pp. 1–15.
Mount, Nick. *Arrival: The Story of CanLit*. House of Anansi, 2017.
Mount, Nick. *When Canadian Literature Moved to New York*. U of Toronto P, 2005.
Munro, Alice. *Lives of Girls and Women*. 1971. Penguin, 2014.
Munsch, Robert. "All about Robert Munsch." *The Official Robert Munsch Site*, https://robertmunsch.com/about. Accessed 29 July 2024.
Munsch, Robert. *Love You Forever*. Firefly Books, 1986.
O'Farrell, Mary Ann. *Telling Complexions: The Nineteenth-Century English Novel and the Blush*. Duke UP, 1997.

Rabin, Roni Caryn, and Azeen Ghorayshi. "Alabama Rules Frozen Embryos Are Children, Raising Questions about Fertility Care." *The New York Times*, 21 Feb. 2024, www.nytimes.com/2024/02/20/health/ivf-alabama-abortion.html.
Ross, Sinclair. *As for Me and My House*. 1941. McClelland & Stewart, 1989.
Rushton, Peter, and Gwenda Morgan. *Banishment in the Early Atlantic World: Convicts, Rebels and Slaves*. Bloomsbury Academic, 2013.
Schneider, Ana-Karina. "Clinging to Flesh: Embodied Experience in Contemporary Women's Dystopias." *Contemporary Women's Writing*, vol. 16, no. 3, May 2022.
Shirm, Gretchen. "Sheila Heti, Melanie Klein and *Motherhood*." *Critique Studies in Contemporary Fiction*, vol. 63, no. 3, May 2022, pp. 309–20.
Skinner, Andrea Robin. "My Stepfather Sexually Abused Me When I Was a Child. My Mother, Alice Munro, Chose to Stay with Him." *Toronto Star*, 7 July 2024.
Statistics Canada. *Fertility in Canada, 1921 to 2022*. Government of Canada, 31 Jan. 2024, www150.statcan.gc.ca/n1/pub/91f0015m/91f0015m2024001-eng.htm.
Stouck, David. *As For Sinclair Ross*. U of Toronto P, 2005.
Stouck, David. "'Introduction: The Reception of *As For Me and My House*'." *Sinclair Ross's 'As For Me and My House': Five Decades of Criticism*, edited by David Stouck, U of Toronto P, 1991, pp. 3–13.
Sugars, Cynthia. "The Anatomy of Influence: Robertson Davies's Psychosomatic Medicine." *Mosaic*, vol. 33, 2000, pp. 72–89.
Thomas, Audrey. *Mrs. Blood*. Talonbooks, 1970.
Warmelink, J. Catja, et al. "Collaboration of Midwives in Primary Care Midwifery Practices with Other Maternity Care Providers." *Midwifery*, vol. 55, Dec. 2017, pp. 45–52.
WHO. "Why We Need to Talk about Losing a Baby." *World Health Organization Newsroom*, www.who.int/news-room/spotlight/why-we-need-to-talk-about-losing-a-baby. Accessed 30 July 2024.
York, Lorraine. *Literary Celebrity in Canada*. U of Toronto P, 2007.

5

DECOLONIZATION AS CURE

Hospitals, Illness, and Healing in Contemporary Indigenous Novels

As Daniel Heath Justice (Cherokee) explains in *Why Indigenous Literatures Matter* (2018), stories can be "agents of both harm and healing" (4). This chapter explores narrative depictions of the impacts of colonialism as a disease to be cured and the healing of Indigenous resurgence.

Indigenous authors in Canada have frequently represented how systemic racism, colonial violence, and the residential school system have caused mental illness and addictions. Depicting the disorders of the settler state, the novels by Indigenous authors discussed in this chapter figure the painful work of decolonization and resurgence as a kind of cure. In Anishnaabe author Richard Wagamese's *Medicine Walk* (2014), a son journeys with his father to understand his history and experiences of addiction. In Métis author Cherie Dimaline's *The Marrow Thieves* (2017), winner of the Governor General's Award for children's literature and the Kirkus Prize for young readers, Indigenous people are hunted for their brains to cure a dream-stealing virus. Cree writer and lawyer Michelle Good's Governor General's Award-winning *Five Little Indians* (2020) traces the trauma of residential school in five survivors' ongoing experiences of mental illness, addiction, and recovery. No kindness or real healing can be found through official medical systems in these novels and the characters instead access cures through experiences that offer hope of decolonization.

The idea of decolonization demands education that centres Indigenous knowledge and experience rather than a monoculture of forms of thought associated with colonial history (see Battiste). In each of these novels, characters find paths to decolonization through learning about traditional knowledge, whether through storytelling in Wagamese's novel, language in

DOI: 10.4324/9781003340119-6

Dimaline's, and medicinal practice in Good's. This education contributes to the characters' sense of healing from colonial harm and permits the novels themselves to represent remedies.

In writing about Indigenous authors to showcase their critiques of this country, its ills, and often-inequitable healthcare system, I acknowledge my own position as the beneficiary of generations of colonial settlement and as a member of a family of doctors trained in Western medicine. My understanding of Indigenous experience and philosophies of healing is necessarily incomplete, and I put forward this chapter not to make definitive claims about reconciliation and the healing of resurgence, but rather as an account of reading fiction to heed and learn from perspectives that have been silenced too long.

From Residential Schools to Carceral Hospitals: Healing Stories and the Ills of Colonialism

Readings of these three novels about intergenerational trauma, the harms of residential schools, and the impact of racism in the Canadian healthcare system should be informed by three crucial contexts: the Truth and Reconciliation Commission of Canada (TRC), Indigenous concepts of healing, and the history of colonial illness and medicine.

Established as part of a legal settlement for survivors, from 2007 to 2015 the TRC sought to document and raise awareness about the widespread, acute, and lasting suffering of generations of Indigenous children who were taken from their parents and forced into residential schools during the nineteenth and twentieth centuries. The TRC's final report describes reconciliation as the quest for greater acknowledgement of the past to benefit relationships of the future (6). Some contest the impact and methods of the TRC (see Green), and the notion of reconciliation itself has been increasingly critiqued (see Gaertner; Turner; Simpson 46–49), but the Commission did increase public knowledge of the devastation of residential schools and other colonial ruptures within Indigenous communities.

Although the idea of reconciliation does not represent a simple remedy or easy progress from a troubled past to a future absolved of responsibility, it does open pathways for non-Indigenous Canadians to better understand their relation to the history and future of Indigenous people and to support Indigenous healing and resurgence. Reading the works discussed in this chapter and assimilating their lessons regarding Canadian healthcare, the trauma of residential schools, and the meaning of healing represents one such step.

The TRC's final report includes ninety-four Calls to Action (319–37), including regarding the duty of the Government of Canada to preserve

Indigenous languages (Calls 13 to 17), and to acknowledge and remediate the ongoing harm to health posed by the legacy of colonial violence and residential schools and by discrimination in the healthcare system (Calls 18 to 24). The novels discussed in this chapter were all published during or since the conclusion of the Commission and can be read in relation to these calls to promote and preserve language and storytelling cultures and to combat healthcare inequities.

These novels also reveal the relationship between health and storytelling, an alignment that is clearer in Indigenous healing practices than in Western medicine. Contemporary scholars across disciplines have often taken up the idea that Indigenous storytelling heals (see for example Adelson and Olding; Dennis and Minor; Neilson; Moura-Koçoğlu). Concepts of the therapeutic power of Indigenous narrative have been most influentially developed in Canada by Jo-Ann Episkenew (Métis) in *Taking Back Our Spirits: Indigenous Literature, Public Policy, and Healing* (2009). Episkenew argues that "Not only does Indigenous literature respond to and critique the policies of the Government of Canada; it also functions as 'medicine' to help cure the colonial contagion by healing the communities that these policies have injured" (2). Jo-Ann Archibald (Stó:lō and St'at'imc) explores the power of Indigenous "storywork" to heal people and communities (85–100), and Armand Garnet Ruffo (Chapleau Fox Lake Cree) cites her work in explaining how the Medicine Wheel can be used as an interpretive model for narrative that incorporates Indigenous ways of knowing. Rather than being a metaphorical way of speaking about the benefits of reading, in this framework narrative is itself medicine—a conduit to cures.

This idea of story is part of a broader understanding of therapeutic methods. Indigenous healing strategies practiced in Canada are diverse with some recurring traits that emphasize the relational nature of the individual, the importance of honouring culture and traditions, and the Medicine Wheel, a four-part understanding of wellness as a physical, mental, emotional, and spiritual balance (Yu et al.). Whereas Western concepts of "medicine" usually imply consuming substances to alleviate symptoms and kill pathogens (see Duffin 94–98), Indigenous healers often "address the disruption by using treatments designed to return mind, body, and spirit to a state of balance" (Methot 192). These novels often dramatize the conflicts between these knowledge frameworks, while showcasing the therapeutic power and meaning of Indigenous concepts of bundles, walking, and storytelling, as well as cedar as a traditional remedy.

It's important to distinguish these depictions of decolonizing healing from the notion of reconciliation, which can imply a relationship with colonial power that may not be welcome. Robyn Green argues that the idea of reconciliation as a cure has been exploited by settler frameworks that underpinned the Truth and Reconciliation Commission. A more helpful concept may be the idea of resurgence, which Leanne Betasamosake Simpson (Michi Saagiig Nishnaabeg) explores in depth and which Aubrey Jean Hanson (Métis) suggests best explains the healing power of literature by Indigenous authors (75). Renate Eigenbrod reads the work of Indigenous stories about Canadian residential schools as acts of "survivance," a concept developed by the Chippewa (Minnesota White Earth) scholar Gerald Vizenor. The decolonizing benefits of storytelling and Indigenous healing practices contribute to survivance and resurgence in these novels.

While residential school experiences appear in this fiction, their intergenerational harms also trouble the characters, from the parenting difficulties faced by survivors to experiences of chronic trauma-induced addiction. As the TRC documented, in addition to physical and sexual abuse, the injuries inflicted by the schools included attacks on relationships, because of isolation and the severing of family ties, and in the damage done to survivors' relational capacities as adults. Part of this cruelty inhered in the destruction of knowledge of Indigenous languages, which contain profound cultural wealth and connect community members to each other and to a sense of kinship across generations (80–84). In the novels discussed in this chapter, this intergenerational colonial trauma impacting the health of relationships is an indicator and cause of physical illness.

Notions of the relationship between colonialism and illness tend to focus on early smallpox epidemics as the key scourge that "emptied" the Americas for Europeans to occupy (Piper 10–11). Yet, as Liza Piper shows, more recent studies demonstrate that this pattern, though it was devastating and widespread (see Daschuk), was neither decisive nor uniform. Many successive waves of various diseases impacted Indigenous populations in North America during early colonial periods, but, as Piper explains, they continued through twentieth-century epidemics of influenza and tuberculosis, and persist now in the ongoing effects of increased rates of diabetes and alcoholism (Jones 19). To the extent that the colonization of the territory now known as Canada is a process of decimation through disease, it is ongoing. David S. Jones points out that, alongside the impact of illnesses themselves, policies that rationalize epidemics as normal and expected for Indigenous populations continue to enforce racist colonial control.

In the context of this history, alcohol addiction, which features prominently in Good and Wagamese's novels, must be understood as one of the illnesses that arrived with colonization and stayed, perpetuating and revealing its effects. Its harm in Indigenous communities has too often been, to use Jones's term, rationalized as inevitable (see Golding). While the condition can be read for its colonial causes, addiction was also used for colonial goals. Until the late twentieth century, policy regarding Indigenous assimilation in Canada leveraged access to alcohol, so that sales to Indigenous people depended on their acquiescence to colonial notions of citizenship (see Campbell). Describing alcoholism itself as a disease is sometimes contested by critics of the "medical model" (Brown 14), which looks for biological causes for suffering that can be treated by Western medicine (Duffin 94–98). Critics of such ways of framing alcoholism complain that it does not sufficiently account for the personal, social, and historical origins or consequences of this substance-use disorder, especially among Indigenous communities (see Johnson; Thatcher). A path forward between the medical model and Indigenous knowledge frameworks is evident in a recent biomedical study conducted in collaboration with Indigenous elders that shows the efficacy of Sweat Lodge ceremonies, a practice that appears in Good's novel, as treatment for substance-use disorder and intergenerational trauma (see Marsh et al.). My readings here proceed with the understanding that, like many colonial illnesses, alcohol addiction often results from and is perpetuated by ongoing systemic harms.

Another important context for this literature is the colonial legacy permeating Canada's public healthcare system, which, despite its reputation, does not offer equal access to care. In *Structures of Indifference* (2018), an influential account of the systemic failures that led to the 2008 death of Brian Sinclair in a Winnipeg emergency room, authors Mary Jane Logan McCallum and Adele Perry expose how racism regularly obstructs care in Canada's often inequitable medical system. They explain that the hospital itself is a key "structure of indifference" that compounds the racism of Canada's healthcare system (62–105). Invoking the work of the philosopher Michel Foucault, Linda Mussell examines the place of the hospital, alongside residential schools and prisons, as one of the carceral institutions subjecting Indigenous people to colonial confinement in Canada. Foucault famously argues that hospitals discipline as well as minister to patients (172–92), and he writes in *Discipline and Punish* (1977) that "the hospital is increasingly conceived of as a base for the medical observation of the population outside" (212). In these novels this outward-looking scrutiny extends from healthcare workers to agents of state control, a link that may be interpreted as a component of Canada's government-managed healthcare system.

State healthcare in the novels discussed here is a coercive force that hardly differs from the injustice of colonial educational institutions. Readers should be alert to how the hospital and the residential school stand as parallel structures in these books, a context McCallum and Perry address (62–63). The history of the impact of health policies on Indigenous people in Canada contains many episodes that can be read for their carceral results. The long-term transfer, for example, of Inuit patients with tuberculosis from Nunavut to Ontario's Hamilton Sanatorium in the 1950s and 1960s is another carceral episode that is too rarely remembered (see Beattie), as are the racist derelictions of care in Canada's segregated "Indian hospitals" of the 1920s to 1980s (see Lux, and Geddes). Indigenous people living in northern communities across the country continue to face greater obligations to travel for treatment, including for cancer (Horrill et al.) and maternity care (Smylie et al.). While some might argue that being obliged to travel for healthcare should not be aligned with imprisonment, even when not forced, such requirements are coercive because they leave Indigenous patients with little choice between survival and admission to distant, often-hostile institutions. Good's characters in particular keep escaping hospitals before they have recovered because hospitals connect them to policing authorities and tend to be places that enforce rather than heal.

The authors discussed in this chapter consider the status of healthcare and repeatedly question what it means to administer medicine. In their novels, public healthcare providers bring both medicine and harm to Indigenous individuals and communities, while the hospital must be read for its function as a colonial structure, much like a residential school. This context, alongside broader notions of Indigenous healing strategies and the lessons of the TRC, should be kept in mind while reading these books.

Richard Wagamese's *Medicine Walk* (2014)

In Richard Wagamese's *Medicine Walk*, a son accompanies his father on a final journey that overcomes their estrangement. The healing of the "medicine walk" may be for Eldon, who seeks atonement as he is dying of alcohol addiction, but also for his son, Franklin, who finds consolation in hearing out his absentee father. Francesca Mussi points out that this access to healing through the land also appears in Wagamese's *Indian Horse* (2012). Dwayne Donald (Beaver Hills Cree) draws a connection between the therapeutic power of walking and the *nêhiyaw* (Cree) concept of *wâhkôhtowin*, an important notion of profound spiritual relatedness that etymologically implies "bent-over walking" to gather from the land (59). This concept illuminates Wagamese's alignment between story, healing, and walking, and his framing of his novel itself as a medicinal journey.

Illness instigates travel in this book but also pushes people to talk as part of a quest for survival. Eldon needs to say his piece before he dies, but Franklin must bring him to a place where his father will tell him the stories he needs to hear. In this sense, the cure of storytelling arrives because of the poison of illness. If pain and illness demand a search for medicines and cures, alcohol seems to promise such relief but brings only more affliction.

This contradiction is a major focus of Wagamese's book and recalls the ancient alignment between "poison" and "cure" in the Greek word "*pharmakon*," which Jacques Derrida famously uses to frame the meaning of writing.

Such issues of interpretation are central to this novel, as when Franklin observes his father carefully and the outline of his face is akin to a drawing that could spell out answers:

> The kid watched him, studying his face and trying to see beyond what he thought he knew of the man, the history that was etched there, the stories, the travels, and after a while all he could see were gaunt lines and hollows and the sag and fall of the skin and muscle and the bone beneath it all.
>
> *(50)*

Wagamese is dramatizing the difficulty of understanding another person, despite proximity and a desire to know, despite biological connection. His father's face both tempts Franklin to interpret the history it contains and resists the effort. Franklin's thwarted desire to understand his father's face as a story reflects the barriers and gateways presented by language itself. This is the same horizon that exists between any caregiver and patient as we have seen in other works from *The English Patient* to *Boy in the Moon*, where the evidence of the body remains as the ultimate signal to be interpreted when language fails.

The detailed attention that this novel pays to the symptoms and progression of terminal alcoholism allows it to be read as a kind of medical case history of the disease. As Becka relates, based on her father's experience with the addiction, "ya gotta drink to stay alive at the same time it's killin' ya" (74). Eldon is "fixin' to die" as the book opens (20), even as "he's been busy dying a long time now" (3). Wagamese offers a clinical account of his symptoms. The illness that has desiccated Eldon's body (14, 16) takes his appetite (78) and words (26), gives him a fever (62), and makes him vomit (234), cough (14), and lie (3). The old man warns Franklin that his father is "gonna be sick" (2) if they walk together. As Franklin says of his father to Becka when they first meet, "He's drink sick. He's dying" (72), because his liver has been destroyed by alcohol (39). Readers should contrast the diagnostic precision of knowing just which organ is failing with the larger ill of facing a life besieged by trauma and systemic racism. At this late stage of illness, Eldon is also drinking because he's so sick (44), and alcohol calms his withdrawal symptoms. Wagamese's characters turn to alcohol because of other pain: we learn that "Eldon got broke up pretty bad inside" (56) and alcohol helps him deal with guilt (200). Eldon connects with Franklin's mother partly because of alcoholism, as she tells him, "I know about the need. . . . Done my share of hurtin' too" (187). In general, as the old man tells Frank, "whisky keeps things away that some people don't want around" (55). This novel displays the circular torment of how pain causes alcoholism, which causes pain.

The characters offer and seek out a variety of medicines for alcoholism, but also for the emotional suffering that prompts addiction. Becka recommends cedar tea for the sickness of alcohol withdrawal (72) and says, "She's an old cure but a good'un" (75), when it helps Eldon's fever. As in *The Marrow Thieves* and *Five Little Indians*, cedar represents an important traditional therapeutic substance. In response to Franklin's question, "You know cures?" (75), Becka explains, "My dad was Chilcotin. My mother was Scotch. They both had heads fulla the old ways" (75). Dual traditions give Becka access to healing insight and knowledge. She gives Franklin a special medicine that she once made for her own father (104–5). When he takes some (111), and it starts to soothe his symptoms, he wants a story (112–13). When the old man who raised him brings Franklin on walks to look for plants, "He called it a medicine walk" (65). Franklin explains that they took these walks because "You gotta spend time gatherin' what you need. What you need to keep you strong" (65). Picking up cures along the way and letting them out as narrative, these characters search the forest for words like medicines and gather stories for strength.

Storytelling offers the most powerful medicine in this novel, and its title—*Medicine Walk*—should be read as referencing the work of narrative. The title positions the act of telling and hearing the story, that is, writing and reading the novel itself, as a therapeutic journey. Eldon explains to Franklin that "I want you to head into the backcountry with me" (21) because "There's things need sayin'" (22), to which Franklin responds, "So you can feel better?" (22). Eldon explains that he wants to take this journey with Franklin because "I got some story that's needed telling for a long time" (80). Since Eldon is taking this journey partly to end his life and be buried in the wilderness (22), Wagamese puts forward the idea that storytelling is a kind of palliative care, the act of telling and listening an end-of-life treatment. As the old man tells Franklin, "folks need hearing out sometimes" (56), while his mother says, "Stories work to calm you down" (191). The interest in talking to heal in *Medicine Walk* can be connected to the Freudian idea of the "talking cure," which Vikki Visvis examines in relation to the work of Haisla and Heiltsuk novelist Eden Robinson. Both Eldon's and Franklin's mothers tell stories at night. After his father's death in the war, his mother reads out loud at night (85, 87, 89, 90). Franklin's mother tells stories at night too (191), because, she says, "they were always in me" (192), a trait that makes her like a "shaman" (192). This repetition of women as nighttime raconteurs positions storytelling as part of their work as caregivers, and contrasts with how Eldon is able to tell his story only in the evening of his own life. Throughout, Wagamese's book raises questions about how women and men talk and tell stories, and how the practice signals and impacts their health.

In his examination of the healing power of story, Wagamese considers the limits of this medicine from a variety of angles, whether of access, willingness, or remembering. As the book opens, Eldon explains to his son that stories are all he has to leave him, to which Franklin responds, "Ain't never gonna be enough" (23). But Wagamese's novel builds a powerful counterargument. Eldon's family name, "Starlight," registers their role as storytellers (159), while Becka concludes that "It's all we are in the end. Our stories" (103). In this book, storytelling is the core feature of identity and a source of healing and solace. While stories come from other people, the characters also draw ideas from looking at ancient rock art (66, 68). Franklin says, "Near as I can figure they're stories," and he feels that these drawings will tell him what he needs to know (69). Wagamese questions whether one can live from such stories (69): Eldon says that "Stories never seemed likely to keep a guy goin'" (69), but Wagamese implies that Franklin disagrees. He studies the drawings, not to translate them precisely, but to learn from their mystery as a kind of therapy that others miss because they have forgotten about the drawings (69). Wagamese also circles the stakes and impacts of silence and forgetting as the opposite of storytelling. Eldon explains that, growing up partly Indigenous, with incomplete traditional knowledge of life on the land, "they learned how to forget about it" (48). Learning to forget was part of his coming of age, and one source of his trauma. Eldon feels that "Stories were his wound. When he came to think of them it wasn't for the glimmer of worlds spun out of darkness and firelight, it was for the sudden holes life can sometimes fall into" (91). For Eldon, "Some stories never need tellin'" (196). When he relates his most traumatic story to Franklin, Becka observes that, "Tellin' you. That took some grit" (102), because most people try to forget instead, "Like forgettin's a cure unto itself" (102). This novel asks whether forgetting or telling of pain offers the better cure.

This book about the medicine of walking and storytelling also considers the meaning of what people carry. Whereas Eldon's best friend Jimmy told him "We carry each other into battle now" (161), after Franklin hears the traumatic story of Jimmy's death in the Korean War, aided at the end by Eldon's own knife (165), he tells his father, "Musta been hard. . . . Carrying Jimmy all this time" (166). After the war, Eldon realized that "Time was a thing he carried" (173). He leaves Franklin's mother with "the feel of her eyes on him what he carried away" (201), while he says that "all's I got left is the story of her now" (217). Memories and stories are also something to carry. When Eldon dies, Franklin brings a stone back from the grave for Bunky, because, he says, "I figured you mighta lost something too" (244). They put it on the hearth so they can "share it, talk of it if we need to" (244). These characters carry memories sometimes as physical objects, sometimes as stories. As they get to know each other, Franklin's mother tells Eldon, "I get that some stories are hard to tell. Like when you heard my story, it took you back to something. To someone, maybe. Back to a story you been carrying a long time" (196). She repeats this formulation as she encourages him to talk. "When you share stories you change things," she says, adding that "If you told me one of your stories, you'd get lighter," and, as a result, "You could let go of something maybe you carried for a long time" (203). Wagamese develops this idea of story as something that people carry and are relieved to put down through narration. As he thinks about his long-dead mother, Franklin wonders if "enough of her spirit had clung to him . . . to carry him forward without loneliness" (232). Carrying her spirit would carry him. Wagamese uses the overlapping potential meanings of "carrying" to explore the restorative and healing impact of story. In this book, stories can be carried, lost, and hidden, as much as physical remnants of the past that endure independent of memory.

Through this painstaking investigation of the healing of story and what it means to carry stories and each other, the idea of the walk serves as an important symbol, while moving itself is part of healing. Eldon asks his son, "The old man teach ya to move through fear?" (111). When Franklin was younger, and mad at his father, he learned that "ya got to move through it" (138). Eldon walks off his feelings as a younger man (206–7), and, after hearing his story, Franklin reflects that "The skeletal man who slept in front of him seemed to resemble nothing of the man who'd walked through the tale he told" (232). When Eldon leaves with Franklin's mother, Bunky gives them a truck because he says he doesn't want her walking and then goes for a walk himself (213). After he tells Bunky about his journey with his father, they go for a final walk (243). This book positions itself as a walk, and walking is its most recurrent and significant gesture. Characters are constantly walking through their stories and trauma, and those who do not are the most lost. At his lowest, for Eldon, "coming and going had become the same direction" and "nowhere was a place he occupied" (173). Franklin observes that, at the start of their final time together, "We're both kinda at the same spot, him'n me" (121). Being always in the same spot is a sign of stalled healing.

For Wagamese, the healing potential of the walk is a broad metaphor that touches on many aspects of the characters' experience. When Eldon finds he wants to go back to Franklin's mother each night, and, thinking about whether he could also return to his own mother, he starts "wonderin' if returnin' was somethin' a man could do, if ya could walk back over your trail and maybe reclaim things" (218). The idea of the walk back opens a view of himself as able to make amends. Bidding farewell to his father's body, Franklin speculates about the final destination of his walk, saying, "I hope when you get to where you're goin' that she's standing there waitin' for you" (238). In a final encapsulation of its study of the healing power of walking, the book closes with Franklin's vision of generations walking through the valley, a dream of a hopeful and healthy lineage and community: "He raised a hand to the idea of his father and mother and a line of people he had never known" (245). Eldon's legacy is to give Franklin some knowledge of himself through story, despite the unknowing in everyone's past and a traumatized habit of trying to forget. The vision of an ancestral community thriving through walking expresses this healing.

The destroyed sense of lineage, history, and connection that drove Eldon to alcohol addiction is partially restored for Franklin through the storytelling of the medicine walk, which offers a kind of cure for the loss of history.

Cherie Dimaline's *The Marrow Thieves* (2017)

In Cherie Dimaline's postapocalyptic novel *The Marrow Thieves*, Indigenous identity is sought and available in dreams, which occupy physical space in the body, and which promise healing. The characters are subject to an industrial scale of dream harvesting that resembles concentration camps and that happens in "schools": Frenchie's father explains that "the Governors' Committee didn't set up the schools brand new . . . they were based on the old residential school system" (5). This historical critique links the theft of dreams to the harms and extractive logic of colonialism, which tends to proceed by seizing resources (see Bernauer; Willow).

Residential schools systematically attacked Indigenous languages by design, so Dimaline's novel considers how language matters to the capacity to dream. As Patrizia Zanella points out, in this novel language is "something that exists in community and that puts speakers in relation to each other" (190). For Paul Huebener, the novel "represents colonization as a conflict between two different cultural models of sleep and dreams" (68). Citing the Potawatomi philosopher Kyle Powys Whyte's influential essay on dystopian Indigenous futures and conservation efforts, in his discussion of Dimaline's novel, Huebener points out the sense of a postapocalyptic present for many Indigenous communities (84), which is reflected in recent discussions of Indigenous literature and culture (see for example, Alter; NoiseCat; Stonechild; TallBear). The novel regards the aftermath of attacks on Indigenous languages and how ancestral language lets dreams both of the past and the future be witnessed, shared, and sustained in a process that proves essential for healing.

Some sense of pre-colonial identity is both desired by the characters, and proves difficult to access, as they seek new methods by which to engage with traditional customs. The protagonist Frenchie explains that "Us kids, we longed for the old-timey. We wore our hair in braids to show it" (21). The reservoir of this sense of identity, these characters find, is not so much in the adoption of a hair style, but available at all times in their biology. Miigwans explains that "We go to the schools and they leach the dreams from where our ancestors hid them, in the honeycombs of slushy marrow buried in our bones" (90). Dreams are the crucial substance preserving Indigeneity. As Sherryl Vint explains, the novel "makes visible the continuity between recent sites of the extraction of biovalue and a longer history of dehumanizing and dispossessing indigenous peoples" (122). This sense of the elixir embedded in bones is not only key to the epidemic Dimaline imagines, but it also underpins the idea of medicine she illustrates. Frenchie describes how being alone in the forest at night reveals "the bleached skeleton of the universe," saying, "This was our medicine, these bones" (9). The night sky reveals the medicine of a universal skeleton: healing depends on a sense of biological identity.

This book's interest in dreams as a biological aspect of the body shows far less dualism than Sheila Heti's in *Motherhood*, for example. Dimaline's book could also be productively read in tandem with Emily St. John Mandel's *Station Eleven*, as both works exhibit characters wandering through broad and changed national landscapes as a result of epidemic illness. Miig references Camus's *The Plague*, describing how it's about "all these people trapped inside their own town because the plague attacks them and they are put into quarantine" (53). In contrast to the entrapment of this most famous epidemic novel, Dimaline and Mandel's contagion books show people spread out and wandering. As they go, in each work characters both stave off and succumb to death from ailments that would have been treatable in the world before the disaster. The works share a sense of longing and melancholy in reflecting the duration of the deprivation of these wandering characters, and the illnesses that they suffer in their postapocalyptic worlds. Rose's sad memory of how her great-uncle fell ill and died after walking for six years (71) could be an incident from *Station Eleven*. Though they both thus share a narrative focus on journeying because of illness, these works differ in important respects. Mandel's novel overlooks Indigenous attachments to the landscape through which her characters travel. Dimaline's work offers a corrective to this oversight. The wandering her Indigenous characters pursue is also to escape a plague, but in her work the epidemic illness is deeply associated with the misappropriations of colonialism and the landscape itself is positioned as already stolen and poisoned by this theft. In their tales of surviving epidemics on colonized land, therefore, these books resemble each other, while their points of contrast help to bring Dimaline's framing of the cures of decolonization into focus.

An atmosphere of pervasive illness haunts Dimaline's novel. When Miig found him he was "half dead, sick from spoiled supplements" (213), and had also long been sick with a cough (14) that was "near constant" (14). Among the group, "Everything was always damp, so we were trained to sniff out mould to keep that sickness at bay" (19). Chronic illness as a result of the physical conditions of the journeying is a constant threat. The group has "No time for sickness" (93), but the wet season brings a serious risk of contagion (93). Most members of the group were sick through the winter, for which "Mineva boiled cedar branches and pine needles into medicine and fed it each of us every two hours" (93). A traditional medicine widely used among Indigenous North American communities (Joseph 91), cedar is also a cure in *Medicine Walk* and *Five Little Indians* (3). For Minerva in particular, the illness "makes her nervous" because a baby she was caring for succumbed to it (93), and Frenchie describes her panic in administering medicines to the group, "as if we were all sick babies she was trying to save" (93). Sickness is a constant condition, threat, and regret.

In Dimaline's book, pain crosses between biology and emotions. Frenchie has "a rotten hole in one of [his] molars" (1), which "screamed every time a swallow of liquid passed over it" (12), while he compares his last sight of his mother's eyes to "the hole in [his] molar, a true ache" (13). Speaking of his mother "stung" and "hurt" (1), while he longs for his "parents as physical pain at the bottom of my stomach and under each kneecap" (139). Just as dreams in this book are biological aspects of the body, physical pain, of teeth, from illness, manifest spiritual and emotional anguish. Characters turn to substances and drugs to alleviate their suffering, and "There were a lot of years where we were lost, too much pain drowned in forgetting that came in convenient packages: bottles, pills" (24). The status of the pill in this context is worth attending to. Though official medical culture often distributes its genuine cures in the form of pills, here, like intoxicating substances, pills often offer stand-ins for cures—a false hope. "The Governors turned to the church and the scientists to find a cure for the missing dreams," Dimaline writes, while those with money sought out pills for sleeping and waking, counselling, and hypnosis (88). Pills offer help with the progress of physical life that should be automatic with good health. The Indigenous marauder who tries to sell the group to the dream thieves is in an "Unnatural state" (133) due to his dependence on unspecified "pills" (136). Even in this terrible instance, when a drug-induced mania seems to cause a child's death (136), the possibility remains that the man's unhealthy dependence is due to the traumas of colonial history. The real source of absolution and a curative effect is a literal path forward: "Once we honored the pain and left it on the side of the road," Miigwans explains, "we moved ahead" (24). The way out of pain is to pay attention to it, and then intentionally leave it behind. Perhaps because sources of healing are present in characters' bones, analgesic effects cannot be accessed through consumption, but rather through pursuing survival from colonial harms.

Dimaline links the historical impacts of smallpox on Indigenous communities to the new plague that has caused the postapocalyptic conditions in which her characters are suffering. At first, Miig explains, Indigenous people won many battles with colonizers, but losing came with new sicknesses. He suggests the colonizers opened the schools because they preferred to keep the Indigenous people as incapacitated as they'd been when "on our knees with fever and pukes" (23). Dimaline draws a direct line between the impact of epidemic illness and the opening of residential schools that further decimated Indigenous communities. The new scourge is a mirror for smallpox in how it devastates Indigenous life at a colonial scale. "Half the population was lost in the disaster and from the disease that spread from too many corpses and not enough graves" (26), Miig explains. "People died in the millions," he says, while the survivors "had to migrate inward. It was like the second coming of the boats, so many sick people and not enough time to organize peacefully" (87). In illustrating this speculative epidemic, Dimaline describes the historical impacts of smallpox in Indigenous communities.

The cure the non-Indigenous officials seek is a kind of pure substance that Indigenous people have been able to keep even as their land was stolen. "Dreams get caught in the webs woven in your bones. That's where they live, in that marrow there" (18), Miigwans explains, continuing, that "You are born with them. Your DNA weaves them into the marrow like spinners" (19). In searching for his husband who has been kidnapped for his dreams, Miig, who has the status of a healer (102), discovers "rows of glass tubes" (144) labelled with Indigenous identities and serial numbers, like the numerical tattoos of Holocaust survivors. He "sang each of them home when I poured them out" (145). Dreams both hearken to Indigenous identity and spirituality but their absence is a version of mental illness, and a reflection of the ongoing nightmare of colonization for these characters.

The missing dream is also the lack of a sense of a future for a landscape too polluted for growth. One of the ills plaguing the world in the lead-up to the apocalyptic dreamlessness is that people "stopped reproducing without the doctors" (26): the fertility treatments that Sheila Heti ruminates over are a harbinger of catastrophe. Dimaline ties the epidemic of dreamlessness itself to the illness of the landscape: "Really the whole world itself got sick" due to climate change, she writes, and the resulting mortality brought a deep, dream-destroying sadness (29). Climate disruption spreads illness, which attacks mental well-being. Frenchie observes, "That's what they were calling the dreamlessness when it started, a plague of madness" (53). This dream-stealing epidemic of mental illness sends its sufferers to medical practitioners seeking cures to be swallowed: "They visited their head doctors—psychiatrists—and they took pills to help them sleep" (29). Even so, Miigwans explains, the disease of dreamlessness worsened, "And a man without dreams is just a meaty machine with a broken gauge" (88). Encapsulated in this memorable depiction is Dimaline's questioning of what makes an enduring identity, what differentiates people from machines.

The antagonists seek to abduct Indigenous people to extract their capacity to dream. "It began as a rumor," Dimaline writes, "that they had found a way to siphon the dreams right out of our bones . . . a rumor denounced every time their doctors sent us to hospitals and treatments centers never to return" (89). The doctors here are agents of the exploitation. As the system grows, Dimaline writes,

> Soon they needed too many bodies, and they turned to history to show them how to best keep us warehoused, how to best position the culling. That's when the new residential schools started growing up from the dirt like poisonous brick mushrooms.
>
> *(89)*

The model for mass exploitation is historical, while the dream-robbing officials promise healthcare only to steal dreams, as "They kept sending us away, enticing us to seek medical care and then keeping us locked up, figuring out ways to hone and perfect their 'solution' for sale" (89). Just as the residential school system promised education but permitted abuse on a massive scale, here the promise of science and healthcare is used to enable exploitation: "They asked for volunteers first. Put out ads asking for people with 'Indigenous bloodlines and good general health' to check in with local clinics for medical trials" (89). The prospect of advancing medicine is used to coerce participants.

The idea of administration is central to this state-sanctioned abuse. Called recruiters, the dream thieves are representatives of national administration and their uniform logo reads "Government of Canada: Department of Oneirology" (4), using the Latin term for the study of dreams. These officials, Dimaline writes, looked to Indigenous people "like the New Agers, looking for ways they could take what we had and administer it themselves" (88). Readers should be alert to the use of the verb "administer" here, a word that travels between healthcare, where treatments are "administered," and legislature, where "the administration" can be a stand-in for the state itself. Furthermore, whereas hospitals administer healthcare, like educational systems, they are also administered by the state: the verb "administer" can indicate coercion as well as care in the power of the state over individuals. Dimaline's book, like Good's, questions what it means to administer in a variety of contexts, and how, even in medical contexts, the state administration of care for Indigenous lives proves difficult to extricate from the brutal legacies of the residential school system. In an environment where administration has historically been violent, the restoration of peace in the concept proves elusive.

The triumph that Dimaline permits her characters over their attackers comes from Minerva's obstruction of the administration of dream theft. "She refused to answer any questions," Dimaline writes, "not that that was integral to the process. All they needed was to insert the probes, tether the wires, and begin the drain" (171). But then she starts humming, and "when the wires were fastened to her own neural connectors. . . . That's when she called on her blood memory" (172). Minerva starts "pulling every dream from her own marrow and into her song" including "words the wires couldn't transfer" (172). Minerva's dreams are in the oldest version of the language (172), and in response "The wires sparked, the probes malfunctioned" (173). As a result, the "school" itself burns down (173), and "the campers made their hands into shallow cups and pulled the air over their heads and faces, making prayers out of ashes and smoke" (174), drawing a ceremony out of the ashes of this place of torture and abuse. In this episode, we can see how Minerva's obstruction of the dream extraction causes the physical infrastructure of the administration to collapse. Stopping the administration of the "treatment" breaks the enforcing administration itself.

Administration and healthcare coincide in Frenchie's discovery of an artifact of his mother's life that his father has managed to preserve despite their long journeying. Frenchie finds a "framed plastic ID card. . . . It was my mother's health card. The green plastic embedded with white letters that spelled out her name" (175). As in Good's *Five Little Indians*, when Lucy becomes a nurse and her daughter aspires to medical school, here the health card can be read as representing how Indigenous people may find their own paths within state-sanctioned medical administration. Nevertheless, that this photographic souvenir of his mother is embedded in the most essential record of Canadian healthcare administration is central to this book's critique of the colonial systems that have legislated, abused, and promised all-too-elusive care to Indigenous people. In considering how Canadians tend to revere their healthcare system, the framed health card should be seen as an under-examined talisman of national culture. Dimaline leaves readers to consider the poignancy of how this most cherished emblem of a pernicious colonial nation is the only physical memento that this Indigenous character has left of his mother.

Administration depends on categories, the boxes to be checked in official forms, but the final hope of escape from the administration, a cure for its ills, comes through characters who transcend such categories and boundaries. Isaac, who speaks the same old Cree that Minerva used to destroy the school and so represents a hope of resurgence (227) is only part Indigenous and trusted the people who kidnapped him because he "didn't have memories in his family of the original schools" that "stayed there, ingesting our children like sweet berries, one after the other, for over a hundred years" (106). The group finds him when they come upon two Guyanese women (223) who "explained that they had been nurses at the Sudbury hospital and saw the treatments and 'volunteer studies' first-hand" and so started rescuing captives (226). Isaac explains how "I was brought into their hospital for blood work to determine my eligibility . . . to make sure my blood wasn't too mixed" (229), and then they "helped me get out of the school" (228). In this instance, in contrast to *Five Little Indians*, hospital staff both permit and facilitate escape, but Dimaline implies that their status both as nurses rather than doctors, hence lower in the hierarchies of authority, and as Black women from the Caribbean, permits their defiance of the hegemonic institutions. The porousness of the identities that administer healing and defy state administration suggest that transcendence is needed for cures.

The landscape and environment have been poisoned in tandem with the spread of the epidemic. Miigwans explains that "The Great Lakes were polluted to muck. It took some doing, but right around the time California was swallowed back by the ocean, they were fenced off, too poisonous for use" (24). At the same time, earthquakes were "peeling the edging off the continents back like diseased gums" (25). During this climate disruption, pipelines snapped "and spewed bile over forests" (87). Closer to coasts the landscape may be healthier, but in the middle of the continent, "It's like where the bomb landed and the poison's leeched [sic] into the banks, everything's gone in all directions" (193). Speaking of a city modeled on Toronto, Frenchie explains that "The smell from the lake here was nauseating. Once this was a popular city, being right on the water. Now this lake, like all the industry-plundered Great Lakes, was poison" (11). This poisoning of the landscape stands in opposition to the idea of medicine and the hope of healing. Clarence explains that "All we need is the safety to return to our homelands. Then we can start the process of healing" (193). Confused, Frenchie asks, "Can't you just heal out here?" (193), to which Clarence responds, "I mean we can start healing the land. We have the knowledge. . . . When we heal our land, we are healed also" (193). Reflecting the theme common to all three of the books discussed here, this notion of healing in the physical landscape as being one with Indigenous resurgence positions decolonization as a cure.

Dimaline's book makes clear that even in a futuristic postapocalyptic vision of Canada, the residential school system still needs burning, while the antidote to its ongoing harms is the transmission of language, history, and stories.

Michelle Good's *Five Little Indians* (2020)

Michelle Good's *Five Little Indians* explores the massive legacy of pain from the characters' experiences in residential school. The book brings readers inside their personal histories, and questions the forms of medicine, pain relief, and cures that they access on their own, or from healers, through organized medicine, and via the judicial system of compensation.

In recounting the stories of five survivors, the book circles the notion of survival itself, with each character positioning their life in relation to the concept. "They call us survivors," Lucy says, but "I don't think I survived" (251). Remembering her friend who died in the school, Clara says "neither of us survived, even though I'm still walking" (198). Later, after she's experienced a healing process in a sweat lodge, Clara feels that "Life was no longer just survival" (199). Showing another angle on the interplay between survival and its opposite, Kenny explains that "Sometimes I think I did die, I'm just still walking around" (255). In urging Howie to participate in the compensation process, Clara acknowledges its challenges but tells him "you've already survived. This is just letting them know what you survived" (278). Good explores survival itself as a liminal state, in which selfhood both endures and keeps suffering from the brutality of the schools. As Good's characters put forward variations on the meaning of survival, she draws attention to the use of this label for the children once held in residential schools. They are called "survivors," but the deep destruction of the system stole something profound about their lives. Good reorients uses of this word into an ongoing question about what it means to survive and the ways in which surviving means continuing to suffer.

One way their survival is not assured is in their ongoing acute pain and distress, which means they are still figuratively struggling to escape the school. For Maisie, who shows Lucy a path forward out of the school but whose young story ends in her suicide, the greatest pain is mental. What she needed, Good writes, was "To be little again, living without fear and brutality—no one gets that back. All that's left is a craving, insatiable empty place" (60). To try to fill the void left as a result of her abuse, Maisie cuts herself, which gives her a feeling of being "clean of pain" (64). For this character, self-harm offers a kind of temporary analgesic, where wounds bring relief. When she re-opens the same wound the next day, she says,

> The second-day pain was not the same. No piercing with the knife. It was duller, but still sharp-enough to make me feel clean. I looked at my face and pressed the wound; the pain sharpened a little and the tension eased.
>
> *(66)*

This character's intense mental distress pushes her to pursue a detailed expertise in the pain relief to be found through the infliction of more pain. The person with whom she pursues abusive sex to appease her trauma gives her a drug that "Made it hard to remember and easy to forget" (70), and on its high, she feels "No pain" (73). The brutality she experienced causes her to seek out toxic varieties of pain relief. When Maisie overdoses on purpose, Good's clinical description of how she "tightened the tubing" around her arm presents a medicalized scene of suicide (78). She ends her story by pursuing the best analgesic drug she's found to its terminal destination, reflecting the scale of the pain that overwhelmed her life.

Whereas Maisie's mental illness proves inescapable, Kenny's agony drives him away from his loved ones, and Lucy suffers from ongoing compulsions. She is constantly "counting the clicks before opening the door" (252), while her daughter calls out her obsessive tallying of the bathroom tiles and multiple rounds of locking and unlocking when she leaves the house, habits that worsen after her father Kenny's intermittent visits (248). Though his unreliability exacerbates her mental distress, Lucy rationalizes Kenny's absenteeism to her daughter by saying she understood that only his pain drove him away (263). Kenny's departures are driven by his suffering. They reflect how many residential school survivors face struggles in their relationships with their children, because, as the TRC explains, they "were denied an environment of positive parenting" (135), leading to further intergenerational harms. Lucy describes how, as a child, Kenny "was not as hollow then as he was now" (106), and says that, if he wasn't an attentive father and partner, "It was himself he couldn't love" (262). Wanting to know why he's interested in the school survivors' lawsuits, Lucy asks "Why pick at the scab?" (253), in a moment that figures his trauma as a physical wound. The anguish of their time in residential school endures in all the characters.

Kenny's body is racked by the pain of illness as well as mental distress. As his liver disease progresses, Kenny has a bath, seeking "a deep heat to soothe the aches and pains that were harder to ignore lately" (249). Since his disease has been caused by alcohol addiction, this pain can be traced back to the emotional injury of being taken from his mother. When he escapes from the school and returns to her, Good writes that the smokehouse where they once spent long happy hours together felt like a "wound" to them both, "a brutal reminder" of Kenny's theft, while relighting its fire feels like a "rebirth" (23). Though they are reunited, the wound can't heal. They don't discuss their time away from each other, which endures "like a silent wound, untended and festering" (23). The breach in their relationship opened a lesion that could never mend. When Kenny asks his mother "Aren't you glad I'm home?" (24), she replies, "I just don't know what to do. . . . It's like most of me is gone and I can't get it back" (25). The pain of these characters stems from how they have all lost crucial pieces of themselves, damaging their capacity to endure.

The characters experience vast suffering for which they seek out a variety of remedies. When Kenny finds his mother again after escaping, he feels "the warmth of her arm around him like medicine" (19). Returning to his mother after the horrors of residential school feels like a chance at a cure. When he gets a coffee at a diner after a rough night, "Kenny downed the first cup like medicine" (247), while Mariah sends Clara out to be with her dog, because, she says, "I can see the medicine between you" (192). Medicine comes in different forms for these characters, but it most frequently arrives through relationships, the loss of which were among the excruciating sources of suffering in residential schools. Recovering in hospital after being horrifically beaten and raped, Howie recounts how the company of his Aunt Mae "was more medicine than what the nurse brought me in a small paper cup" (241). Likewise, while enjoying the summer warmth in contrast to the cold years he spent in prison, Howie finds that "his body remembered the healing heat of his time in the Southwest after his mom had run with him across the border" (276). The heat heals because it's reminiscent of time spent with his mother. Medicine for these characters is found in meaningful relationships.

Alcohol in contrast offers a toxic and addictive analgesic. The alcoholism from which Kenny and his mother suffer arises in direct response to their pain as a result of the residential school system's abuses. "I thought I would die without you," his mother tells him in their first embrace (19), reflecting the massive physical impacts of his theft. Yet it is in this close physical proximity to his mother "that he smelled it for the first time—that sickly sweet smell" (19). This "sickly" scent is the tell of his mother's alcohol addiction, the disease that has arrived with her sorrow at his theft and absence. This description of the "sickly sweet smell" of booze arrives again in Kenny's last chapter, as he's dying from the same illness (245). He is "wishing for a drink" while reading an article about survivors suing the government (252). While his memories of the school caused his alcohol dependency, reading about a chance at retribution spurs his desire to drink. Good shows that re-victimization can occur even in the pursuit of justice. Throughout her narrative, alcohol addiction appears as an illness that happens when characters cannot find the right medicine for their suffering.

Despite their trauma, some of Good's characters find healing in memories, sometimes literally figured in bags and pouches that risk being permanently lost in the physical world. Whereas the morphine for pain a hospital doctor gives Clara sends her into "oblivion" (152–53), the healing that Mariah offers her involves carrying memories along. Clara often touches "the medicine bag Mariah had placed around her neck that first time she went into the lodge" (218). Clara finds enduring solace in keeping this small sack close to her. In contrast, Maisie's doom seems sealed when she loses the bag that held some favourite things and "the only picture I had of my mom" (72). It contains the sense of self that she'd kept beyond the reach of her abuser at school: "I lost sight of the bag, and with it my life as something other than what Father had made me" (72–73). Good leaves open two implications here, either that Maisie loses the bag because she is in a now-inevitable downward spiral, or that losing the bag seals her fate by destroying her last hope at retaining a free feeling of selfhood. Either way, watching as a sense of herself vanishes along with the bag, she says, "It slipped out of me, gone" (73). Readers should attend to the transference Good enacts in describing a bag that is external to this character containing something that slips "out" of her as she loses it. Like the medicine pouch Clara wears, Maisie's bag represents an example of a bundle, an important concept in Indigenous knowledge frameworks (Wemigwans 34–35) and poetics (Scofield, "Poems as Healing Bundles," 318–19). Whether kept or lost, these bundles represent characters' chances at self-sustaining healing, a more abiding and curative medicine than alcohol, street drugs, or doctors' treatments.

The abnegation of care at the schools is part of their attack on the Indigenous characters, an injury that medical professionals keep furthering. The characters often encounter healthcare workers and enter hospitals. When Lucy lands in hospital after falling ill with bronchitis (211), she is eventually discharged with an admonishment to seek medical help earlier next time (215). As Kenny nears death, he awakes with a familiar pain, for which "his doctor had scolded Kenny, telling him his liver couldn't take much more" (251). Doctors and nurses in this book always scold: Good's characters have consistently punishing relations with healthcare providers because they are representatives of a hostile national system that has used the full force of its administration against their lives, families, and well-being.

In the Canadian context, where healthcare is closely aligned with government services and national culture, the hospital system becomes a manifestation of state power. In Good's book, access to this profession and its power is patrolled by its white purveyors, who use arbitrary decrees to keep Good's Indigenous characters out. Lucy enrolls in a training program to become a nurse (104–7), but she is forced to drop out when she becomes pregnant because staying would be "unseemly" (123). Her state is discovered when she experiences nausea while working, and the nurse in charge sends her to see a doctor, telling her that "of course" she won't be able to continue her training (123). Even in this realm of feminized caregiving, where Lucy's "diagnosis" is clear, the nurse in charge still opts to direct her towards the masculinized field with greater official authority by referring her to a physician, telling her to "head off to the maternity ward and I will send a doctor" (123). Not only does she use her power to take away Lucy's chance at self-determination through a career, she further subjects her to the unasked-for attention of a male disciplinary figure, undermining her right to privacy since she doesn't ask Lucy for consent. Struggling with her objections, "Lucy focused instead on Mrs. Reynold's kindness" (123). Good's framing of Lucy's insistence on viewing the nurse as kind reflects the cruel irony at the heart of Indigenous experiences with healthcare professionals in this book: those given official authority to care and heal often perpetuate Indigenous suffering. At best the doctors and nurses diagnose—liver failure, pregnancy—but they do not heal.

Enforcing the disciplinary role the medical system gives them, healthcare providers collude with officials taking action against the Indigenous characters. Waking up in hospital after violent abuse (239), Howie's aunt visits and tells him that he will need to return to the school before he can be liberated because "The nurses will call the police if we take you from here" (240). Healthcare providers serve as agents whose primary allegiance is to a punishing system of authority, rather than to their patients' healing. While in hospital after giving birth to Kendra, Lucy starts to cry on a visit with Clara, because "The welfare lady was here today. She said I have to prove I'm a fit mother" (125). This intrusion happened because, Lucy thinks, "Maybe the nurses called her. I don't know. Maybe they do that to all Indians" (125). Nurses seem a direct conduit to state agents. Afraid officials may take the baby, the women flee the hospital with baby Kendra (125–26). Clara reassures Lucy that no one will look for them, "And besides, I gave them a fake address when I signed you into the hospital" (127). In the official records of medical authority, safety comes from being hidden by false information.

Good's characters often flee hospitals, and these departures should be seen as mirroring the escape from residential school that is her primary focus. When Clara is hospitalized after sustaining an injury while delivering guns to American Indigenous activists, police come "sniffin' around" (151), and George believes that "the hospital must have called them" (151). Hospital-based representatives of official culture collude with the police and other disciplinary figures. While she's still in hospital, "Some guy in a white coat" arrives and "grab[s] Clara's wrist and read[s] her name tag," making her feel "the way she had when they called her number at the Mission" (151). Such brusque impersonal treatment by the doctor immediately re-traumatizes her, showing how a forced stay in a hospital may be experienced as having little difference from incarceration in a residential school, and touch without consent can feel the same in medical environments or in manipulative "educational" ones. After the police visit her in bed (153), once more Clara escapes a hospital, this time with George's help (155), recalling her earlier flight with Lucy and Kendra. These escapes echo the characters' departures from residential school. Readers should be alive to the repetition of these escapes and instances where doctors or nurses either call or are suspected of calling authorities whose objectives are not aligned with their patients' interests. Doctors and nurses, rather than being healers in this text, are representatives of coercive, cruel, and disciplinary administrative regimes.

The escape from the hospital permits these characters to access medicine, healing, and growth that will help them minister to if not fully dissipate their childhood wounds. While the representatives of hospital medicine are untrustworthy, Mariah stands as a healer who operates from beyond the oppressions of colonialism. When she slips out of the hospital, Clara is delivered to "Old Mariah's place" (162) by a distributed network that knows where she can access care that will help. Vera says of Mariah, "She'll doctor you up, take care of you till you're well again" (162). The use of the word "doctor" as a verb rather than a noun is telling, as Mariah is not a credentialed "doctor," but is better at caring than the officially trained physicians whom Good depicts. As Clara says, there was "something calming about Mariah" (190), and she reminds Kendra in the prologue that "Mariah's a doctor, too" (2). Still, Clara feels a residual learned suspicion of traditional healing, remembering that the residential school nun would call an Indigenous healer a "Witch doctor" (190). When it becomes clear that Clara's wound is infected, "Panic start[s] rising in her" and she asks whether she should find a hospital (191). Despite the betrayals of organized medicine, the illness of infection and her colonial inculcation in the residential school makes Clara feel she should seek out such care.

Yet Mariah's cures work, and Good offers a close focus and almost clinical eye on the lineage that has certified her as a healer, and on the techniques of her practice. Explaining why she has access to this traditional medicinal knowledge, Mariah says, "My grandmother raised me here. Hid me. Kept me out of the Indian Schools" (190). She descends through a line of continuity beyond residential schools. Not only did she evade their brutality and thefts of culture, but she also learned traditional healing methods. "My mother died of the coughing sickness," Mariah explains, "so my father brought me here, to my grandmother. . . . She was a healer" (190). Mariah thus represents a female lineage of healers who have transmitted their knowledge beyond the reach of colonial systems that have brought so many ills to their community. The traditional locale of healing that Mariah has established in her home stands in contrast to the hospitals Good portrays, which purport to distribute healing but more often expose their patients to state control. Mariah's way of offering care has its own administrative methods to allow for healing visits, and a payment structure to keep Mariah's work sustainable: "People come here pretty regular," Mariah explains, and, as compensation, "Some bring meat if they've had a good hunt" (190). Recalling the ethical framework for payment preferred by the midwives in McKay's *The Birth House*, here the healer's compensation is optional and based on offerings in kind rather than cash or barter.

Good relays the educational lineage and practicalities that make Mariah's care possible, but she also focuses with textbook precision on her medicinal procedures. Mariah tends to Clara's wound, makes a poultice (191), and removes the bandage, "leaving the infected wound exposed" (191). While this telling focuses the reader on Mariah's care and expertise, the exposures of this deliberate process also offer a metaphor for the painful work of storytelling about the trauma of residential schools, peeling back the bandage to uncover the source of the illness. Good dwells on Mariah's techniques, detailing her ministrations with a clinical eye: she "carefully selected the items" to be boiled for her medicine, "wrapped and tied the package carefully," then "dipped a clean cotton swab in the amber liquid" after the ingredients had steeped, and "gently cleaned the wound," and then "re-bandaged the shoulder" (192). This close visual focus on a traditional healing practice is a form of reverence, tribute, and preservation. Good thus positions this part of her storytelling as a kind of educational text, thereby leveraging the scope of the genre of the novel, which, as the Russian literary theorist Mikhail Bakhtin influentially demonstrates, both parodies and incorporates other genres into itself (5). Just as Dimaline's book questions the meaning of administration, Good's focus on Mariah's traditional healing techniques ponders the stakes and meaning of administering care. Mariah's procedures are effective, and her medical practice that operates from beyond colonial systems brings about a cure for Clara. Mariah heals Clara's wounded shoulder (200), and Good's telling of this episode stands as a kind of case study of traditional medicinal skill. Recalling the "problem-based learning" narratives that are common in medical education and textbooks (see Cumming), this story represents an opportunity for learning.

With her physical wound healed, Mariah also uses traditional techniques to treat Clara's mental well-being. Describing her home, Mariah says, "Like I said before, this is a healing place" (192), and she spends time in the sweat lodge behind her house (193), another therapeutic place that stands in contrast to the hospital. When asked to prepare an offering for the sweat lodge, Clara asks, "Do I have to?" (195), but a younger woman explains that the request is an honour and offers to help her (196), showing how the learning and the transmission of cultural knowledge is part of healing as well as the process of decolonization. As Clara confronts her trauma in the sweat lodge, she recalls the death of her childhood friend Lily from untreated illness at the school. Once more she remembers "how Lily had hemorrhaged to the brink of death in front of her. How Sister Mary had let her die, alone and helpless" (198). Good foregrounds how language and narration are imperfect tools for expressing subtle, complex, and acute perceptions, writing of Clara's experience that "There are no English words to describe how one woman walked into that lodge and another walked out" (199). The healing treatment of Clara's mental distress in the sweat lodge defies simple explanation in the language of the colonizers.

Mariah's treatments are ones Clara can carry with her and share. When she leaves Mariah's place, she takes "medicines" with her (200), and Mariah offers Cree prayers and sage smoke (201), bidding her farewell, saying, "Remember, this is a place of healing. . . . When things get tough, remember the medicine" (203). In contrast to a hospital as a "place of healing," the benefit of Mariah's home is partly as an empowering memory, and in that sense, Mariah's patients can carry her cures with them figuratively as well as literally. Clara makes use of the improvement in her mental well-being by becoming a representative of the "Native Courtworkers' Society" (222), a role that lets her support Howie (227). He credits his employment to her impact, because before his "head was still in prison" and he'd been "feeling desperate when [he] really didn't need to" (227). The fact that Clara's mental health has improved lets her help others in her community, showing the ripple effect of decolonizing treatments among these characters.

All the characters are looking for remedies and cures for their pain, and each finds a different path towards their goal, with the judicial process of compensation offering one imperfect avenue. Just as this novel compares hospitals to residential schools as colonial structures, it also questions the extent to which the judicial system of compensation approximates healing, asking whether a state system and its notions of reconciliation can ever offer a cure for Indigenous trauma. The question is germane for Good, who for more than a decade worked as a lawyer advocating for residential school survivors (Good, "Biography").

Judicial process in this book stands as an equally dubious counterpart to medical process, yet one that in some ways offers more curative hope. Though she supports Kenny as he engages with the process (256), Lucy is at first suspicious of the pursuit of compensation, warning that "It just stirs up a lot of hurtful memories" (251). In his final days, Good shows Kenny circling forms of relief, as, after a night of drinking, opening a window "was an immediate, if incomplete, remedy" (245), and later "The smell of fresh linen was like a remedy" (251). After Kenny speaks to a lawyer about his experiences to start the compensation process, he rushes to the washroom before vomiting, and as he struggles to account for the lawyer's probing questions, he's returned to memories of his abuser, and the pain in his liver overlaps with "all those days of shallow breathing, avoiding the pain of broken ribs" (256). This sequence is a crucial encapsulation of Good's multifaceted exploration of the pain and illness inherent in the trauma of residential school survivors. Relaying his experiences to the lawyer, the representative of the official process, makes Kenny so nauseated that he vomits, yet it also returns him to the scenes of sexual harm he suffered, accentuates his liver pain, and recalls the torture of living with bones broken by an abuser. Two forms of illness in the present, two forms of violent pain from the past, are all being concurrently suffered by this character in one overburdened and excruciating moment as a direct result of dredging his memories for the compensation process. Readers should note how precisely Good delineates the depth of this character's suffering in this palimpsest of agony.

Even with this layering of pain, Good leaves open the possibility that Kenny's acute physical reaction to his interview with the lawyer was a kind of remedy. Vomit is a powerful symbol in literature, and such expulsions from the body may represent duress that obstructs a character's life, purging that offers healing and cathartic effects, or, as Julia Kristeva most famously explores, vomit can be interpreted as an abject counterpart to language, identity, and storytelling itself (3). Good leaves her readers to consider whether Kenny's final illness because of speaking with the lawyer represents an ultimate injury, release, or cure, or simply whether having told his story once, even though the compensation process is not complete, gives him a chance to stop surviving. We can interpret Kenny as throwing up because, like an emetic toxin, the story he has told is incompatible with health, and it can't be kept down any longer. In the most supernatural moment in the book, Kenny awakes the next morning with a perspective on his world from beyond death. He says, "I know I drank myself into a hole last night" (257), but for once his pain "is gone" (257). Though reliving the horror of his experience for the lawyer seems to hasten Kenny's death by pushing him to heavy drinking, he's finally free from pain. Kenny's time with the lawyer may represent another experience of deadly harm, or telling his story may permit a release of his soul. Good leaves open the possibility that both scenarios are true, that the experience offered Kenny both harm and release, showing the complexity of this narrative.

Whereas Kenny can be read as suffering terminal harm from engaging with the compensation process, Howie sees it through and finds it beneficial. "It's not even the money" he tells Clara: "It's about telling my story. Having my say after all these years. Not just me, but for the ones who can't speak out" (273). Reflecting the concept of the benefits of talk therapy (see Scull 203–18), telling the story is not simply the prerogative of survivors, it also contributes to people's ability to thrive as well as survive, and can be part of a healing process.

To the extent that characters heal through therapeutic experiences or compensation, the experience often restores their sense of ownership of the narrative of their own lives as children. As she contemplates whether to pursue a life with Howie, Clara revisits Mariah, and goes into the sweat lodge to try to dispel horrible memories (284). When she feels nothing is working, Mariah tells her to be patient, saying, "Let the healing come to you in its own way" (285). Finally her childhood friend Lily comes to her again in a dream, this time "glowing, bursting with good health" (285), and says, "You cared for me, protected me, held me when the sickness was taking me" (285). While Lily directs her not to suffer from guilt or regret, Clara sees "herself too as a child, glowing with the same radiant health" (285). The experience of healing restores both girls as children in Clara's mind. Lily's visit in the dream is itself a cure, but the vision too shows these girls as cured, healthy at last. Though Lily died, and Clara has always carried the wound, in a kind of resurrection, "now when she thought of Lily, she saw a chubby girl in the bright sun" (291). This healing restoration of stolen childhood reflects Howie's feelings about the ultimate benefits of the compensation process. When he finds out about the money he'll receive, Howie says, "Can't give me back my childhood, but maybe we can make a better life with this" (289). The restoration of a childhood bursting with health and happiness is only possible in visions, but the compensation is a start at atonement.

Justice system workers are counterparts to healthcare workers here, representatives of a colonial system who have an opportunity to help Indigenous communities as well as harm them. Whereas Clara becomes a courtworker, and so represents the empowerment of bringing Indigenous perspectives into the system, Lucy by the same token becomes a nurse, contributing to decolonizing healthcare. In both arenas of state process, health and the law, these women's stories represent the hope that Indigenizing the system could bring about justice. The characters restore a sense of themselves beyond their abuse through the restorations of traditional medicine and the cures of decolonization.

Though Clara pursues a profound sense of healing through multiple experiences with Mariah, of all the characters, Lucy has the most exposure to organized medicine. She has a baby via a caesarian section (121) and becomes so sick with bronchitis that she is hospitalized (211). As Clara writes to Kenny to urge him home to look after his family, Lucy's "fever was so high she almost died" but she hadn't gone to the hospital earlier because she wouldn't leave her daughter (211). Learning of Lucy's sickness persuades Kenny to make a rare return (211): illness brings him back. While Lucy experiences these difficult encounters with the medical system, she also aspires to become a nurse. After she passes her high school equivalency test, she points out a clipping about Indigenous nursing grads, and says, "Look, those Indian girls became nurses. If they can do it, so can I" (104). While Lucy eventually fulfills her goal of becoming a nurse (223), her daughter also aspires to enter the medical profession. As the book closes, Kendra has embarked on a college education with plans to go to medical school (266), and the prologue suggests she becomes the "first Indian doctor in Canada" (2). Although Allan Sherwin suggests that two Indigenous men graduated from Ontario medical schools in the 1860s (20–21), the first Indigenous woman to graduate from the University of British Columbia's medical school was Nadine Caron in 1997 ("Nadine"), a timeline that roughly tracks with Kendra's implied chronology. In general, Indigenous physicians continue to be severely underrepresented in Canada (see Sadler et al. 2–3; D'Hont et al.). Kendra's barrier-breaking path into the practice of medicine cements Good's alignment between the escape from residential school and Indigenous infiltration of a discriminatory public healthcare system.

Whereas Lucy entered the healthcare industry as a nurse, in a generational progression, her daughter takes the further step of achieving even greater authority and prestige in the profession by becoming a physician, a role historically most accessible to white men. Readers should observe the parallel here between Mariah's learning of Indigenous healing traditions from her grandmother in a lineage that remained separate from colonial erasures of knowledge in the residential school system. She represents a female lineage of traditional healers, while Lucy and Kendra represent another line of women healers working from within the colonial healthcare system that so often betrays Indigenous characters. Just as Clara helps Howie by operating within the court system, Good ends her book with the intimation that Lucy and Kendra represent an ongoing hope of Indigenizing and decolonizing the Canadian healthcare system—a key goal of the Truth and Reconciliation Commission of Canada.

Conclusion

When Good's prologue closes and the book begins in earnest, Clara, Lucy, and Kendra enter the sweat lodge for a ceremony to honour the return and burial of Lily's body, with Clara telling Kendra, "Get ready for some doctoring" (3). As "the helpers closed the door" (3) on the women inside the sweat lodge, readers turn the page to open the novel: Good thus positions her story as a medicinal dream that could offer a healing corrective to colonial viewpoints on Indigenous suffering.

Throughout this process, as in the other two novels discussed here, the education in traditional knowledge that represents decolonization offers a hope of healing and a wide variety of cures, whether of the injuries of institutional control, physical suffering and sickness, or the lasting mental trauma of colonial harm. The institution of the hospital, a counterpart to prison, residential school, and the colonial state, represents a site that Indigenous characters both escape and infiltrate. The prospect of decolonization, pursued through generational change, compensation, atonement through storytelling, and the sharing of uncolonized healthcare knowledge, promises healing and cures.

The placement of this chapter about healing at the close of this book about malady has been intentional, as illness implies the wish for cure, and the harms and sicknesses of colonialism represent a tragic source of disorder in the meaning of Canadian culture. In this context, the hope for decolonization as a cure is unending, a constant effort rather than a final destination. Likewise for non-Indigenous Canadians, the idea of reconciliation understood as the work of increasing understanding of the past to forge better relationships for the future is an ever-present goal. As the TRC points out, although Indigenous-only cultural spaces are also essential (281), "Sharing intercultural dialogue about history, responsibility, and transformation through the arts is potentially healing and transformative for both Aboriginal and non-Aboriginal peoples" (280). Readers of Indigenous authors join in resurgence and open new doors with each first page they turn—because narrative can heal.

Works Cited

Adelson, Naomi, and Michelle Olding. "Narrating Aboriginality On-Line: Digital Storytelling, Identity and Healing." *The Journal of Community Informatics*, vol. 9, no. 2, Nov. 2012.

Alter, Alexandra. "'We've Already Survived an Apocalypse': Indigenous Writers Are Changing Sci-Fi." *New York Times*, 16 Aug. 2020.

Archibald, Jo-Ann. *Indigenous Storywork: Educating the Heart, Mind, Body, and Spirit*. U of British Columbia P, 2008.

Bakhtin, Mikhail. *The Dialogic Imagination*. 1981. Translated by Caryl Emerson and Michael Holquist. Edited by Michael Holquist, U of Texas P, 2004.

Battiste, Marie. *Decolonizing Education*. Purich, 2013.
Beattie, Samantha. "Inuit Elders Retrace Steps to Hamilton Sanatorium Where as Children They Endured Traumatic Isolation." *CBC News*, 26 July 2023.
Bernauer, Warren. "The Limits to Extraction: Mining and Colonialism in Nunavut." *Canadian Journal of Development Studies*, vol. 40, no. 3, July 2019, pp. 404–22.
Brown, Brian. "The Health Humanities, Genealogies of Health Care, and the Consolation of Understanding: Towards a Critique of 'Recovery' in Mental Health." *The Routledge Companion to Health Humanities*, edited by Paul Crawford et al., Routledge, 2023, pp. 11–18.
Campbell, Robert A. "Making Sober Citizens: The Legacy of Indigenous Alcohol Regulation in Canada, 1777–1985." *Journal of Canadian Studies*, vol. 42, no. 1, Jan. 2008, pp. 105–26.
Cumming, Allan. "Stories in Medical Education and Training." *Storytelling in Medicine*, edited by Colin Robertson et al., 2nd ed., CRC, 2024, pp. 95–108.
Daschuk, James W. *Clearing the Plains: Disease, Politics of Starvation, and the Loss of Aboriginal Life*. U of Regina P, 2013.
Dennis, Mary Kate, and Michael Minor. "Healing through Storytelling: Indigenising Social Work with Stories." *British Journal of Social Work*, vol. 49, no. 6, June 2019, pp. 1472–90.
Derrida, Jacques. "Plato's Pharmacy." *Dissemination*, translated by Barbara Johnson, U of Chicago P, 1981, pp. 61–120.
D'Hont, Thomsen, et al. "Breaking Trail in the Northwest Territories: A Qualitative Study of Indigenous Peoples' Experiences on the Pathway to Becoming a Physician." *International Journal of Circumpolar Health*, vol. 81, no. 1, July 2022, pp. 1–6.
Dimaline, Cherie. *The Marrow Thieves*. Cormorant, 2017.
Donald, Dwayne. "We Need a New Story: Walking and the *wâhkôhtowin* Imagination." *Journal of the Canadian Association for Curriculum Studies*, vol. 18, no. 2, Mar. 2021, pp. 53–63.
Duffin, Jacalyn. *History of Medicine: A Scandalously Short Introduction*. 3rd ed., U of Toronto P, 2021.
Eigenbrod, Renate. "'For the Child Taken, for the Parent Left Behind': Residential School Narratives as Acts of 'Survivance'." *English Studies in Canada*, vol. 38, no. 3–4, 2013, pp. 277–97.
Episkenew, Jo-Ann. *Taking Back Our Spirits: Indigenous Literature, Public Policy, and Healing*. U of Manitoba P, 2009.
Foucault, Michel. *Discipline & Punish*. 1977. Translated by Alan Sheridan, Vintage Books, 1995.
Gaertner, David. *The Theatre of Regret: Literature, Art, and the Politics of Reconciliation in Canada*. U of British Columbia P, 2020.
Geddes, Gary. *Medicine Unbundled: A Journey through the Minefields of Indigenous Health Care*. Heritage House, 2017.
Golding, Corbin William. "A Prairie Polyphemus: The Firewater Myth in a Canadian Legal Context." *Saskatchewan Law Review*, vol. 86, no. 1, 2023, pp. 1–40.
Good, Michelle. "Biography." *Michelle Good the Writer*, www.michellegood.ca/biography.htm. Accessed 18 July 2024.
Good, Michelle. *Five Little Indians*. Harper Perennial, 2020.
Green, Robyn. "Unsettling Cures: Exploring the Limits of the Indian Residential School Settlement Agreement." *Canadian Journal of Law and Society*, vol. 27, no. 1, Apr. 2012, pp. 129–48.
Hanson, Aubrey Jean. "Reading for Reconciliation? Indigenous Literatures in a Post-TRC Canada." *English Studies in Canada*, vol. 43, Oct. 2018, pp. 69–90.

Horrill, Tara C., et al. "Access to Cancer Care among Indigenous Peoples in Canada: A Scoping Review." *Social Science & Medicine*, vol. 238, no. 112495, Oct. 2019.
Huebener, Paul. "Stealing Sleep: Expanding the Conversation on the Literary Politics of Sleep and Insomnia." *English Studies in Canada*, vol. 44, no. 3, 2018, pp. 67–89.
Johnson, Harold. *Firewater: How Alcohol Is Killing My People (and Yours)*. U of Regina P, 2016.
Jones, David S. *Rationalizing Epidemics*. Harvard UP, 2009.
Joseph, Leigh. *Held by the Land: A Guide to Indigenous Plants for Wellness*. Wellfleet, 2023.
Justice, Daniel Heath. *Why Indigenous Literatures Matter*. Wilfrid Laurier UP, 2018.
Kristeva, Julia. *Powers of Horror*. 1982. Translated by Leon S. Roudiez, Columbia UP, 2024.
Lux, Maureen K. *Separate Beds: A History of Indian Hospitals in Canada, 1920s–1980s*. U of Toronto P, 2016.
Marsh, Teresa Naseba, et al. "The Sweat Lodge Ceremony: A Healing Intervention for Intergenerational Trauma and Substance Use." *International Indigenous Policy Journal*, vol. 9, no. 2, Apr. 2018, pp. 1–22.
McCallum, Mary Jane Logan, and Adele Perry. *Structures of Indifference: An Indigenous Life and Death in a Canadian City*. U of Manitoba P, 2018.
Methot, Suzanne. *Legacy: Trauma, Story, and Indigenous Healing*. ECW, 2019.
Moura-Koçoğlu, Michaela. "To Carry Pain, to Heal through Ceremony: Indigenous Women's Standpoint in Indigenous Australian and Canadian Literatures." *Studies in Canadian Literature*, vol. 48, no. 1, 2023, pp. 169–88.
Mussell, Linda. "Decolonizing Research on the Carceral in Canadian Political Science." *Canadian Journal of Political Science*, vol. 56, no. 3, Sept. 2023, pp. 571–95.
Mussi, Francesca. "Land and Storytelling: Indigenous Pathways towards Healing, Spiritual Regeneration, and Resurgence." *The Journal of Commonwealth Literature*, vol. 58, no. 3, Sept. 2023, pp. 660–76.
"Nadine Caron, MD 97, the First Aboriginal Woman to Graduate from the UBC Faculty of Medicine." *Give UBC*, U of British Columbia, 27 Sept. 2011, https://give.ubc.ca/impact-stories/nadine-caron-md-97/.
Neilson, Shane. "Contrasting Epistemologies: Biomedicine, Narrative Medicine and Indigenous Story Medicine." *Journal of Evaluation in Clinical Practice*, vol. 30, no. 5, Aug. 2023, pp. 741–48.
NoiseCat, Julian Brave. "How to Survive an Apocalypse and Keep Dreaming." *The Nation*, June 2020.
Piper, Liza. *When Disease Came to This Country: Epidemics and Colonialism in Northern North America*. Cambridge UP, 2023.
Ruffo, Armand Garnet. "Exposing the Poison, Staunching the Wound: Applying Aboriginal Healing Theory to Literary Analysis." *The Canadian Journal of Native Studies*, vol. 29, no. 1/2, Jan. 2009, pp. 91–110.
Sadler, Kathy, et al. "Indigenous Student Matriculation into Medical School: Policy and Progress." *International Indigenous Policy Journal*, vol. 8, no. 1, Jan. 2017, pp. 1–15.
Scofield, Gregory. "Poems as Healing Bundles." *Indigenous Poetics in Canada*, edited by Neal McLeod, Wilfrid Laurier UP, 2014, pp. 311–19.
Scull, Andrew. *Desperate Remedies: Psychiatry's Desperate Quest to Cure Mental Illness*. Belknap, 2022.

Sherwin, Allan L. *Bridging Two Peoples: Chief Peter E. Jones, 1843–1909*. Wilfrid Laurier UP, 2012.
Simpson, Leanne Betasamosake. *As We Have Always Done: Indigenous Freedom through Radical Resistance*. U of Minnesota P, 2017.
Smylie, Janet, et al. "Long-Distance Travel for Birthing among Indigenous and Non-Indigenous Pregnant People in Canada." *Canadian Medical Association Journal*, vol. 193, no. 25, June 2021, pp. E948–55.
Stonechild, Blair A. *Challenge to Civilization: Indigenous Wisdom and the Future*. U of Regina P, 2024.
TallBear, Kim. "Indigenous Genocide and Reanimation, Settler Apocalypse and Hope." *Aboriginal Policy Studies*, vol. 10, no. 2, Feb. 2023, pp. 93–111.
Thatcher, Richard W. *Fighting Firewater Fictions: Moving Beyond the Disease Model of Alcoholism in First Nations*. U of Toronto P, 2004.
Truth and Reconciliation Commission of Canada. *Honouring the Truth, Reconciling for the Future: Summary of the Final Report of the Truth and Reconciliation Commission of Canada*. Truth and Reconciliation Commission of Canada, 2015.
Turner, Dale. "On the Idea of Reconciliation in Contemporary Aboriginal Politics." *Reconciling Canada: Critical Perspectives on the Culture of Redress*, edited by Jennifer Henderson and Pauline Wakeham, U of Toronto P, 2013, pp. 100–15.
Vint, Sherryl. *Biopolitical Futures in Twenty-First-Century Speculative Fiction*. Cambridge UP, 2021.
Visvis, Vikki. "Beyond the 'Talking Cure': The Practical Joke as Testimony for Intergenerational Trauma in Eden Robinson's 'Queen of the North'." *Studies in Canadian Literature*, vol. 29, no. 2, June 2004, pp. 37–61.
Vizenor, Gerald Robert. *Survivance: Narratives of Native Presence*. U of Nebraska P, 2008.
Wagamese, Richard. *Medicine Walk*. 2014. McClelland & Stewart, 2019.
Wemigwans, Jennifer. *A Digital Bundle: Protecting and Promoting Indigenous Knowledge Online*. U of Regina P, 2018.
Whyte, Kyle Powys. "Our Ancestors' Dystopia Now: Indigenous Conservation and the Anthropocene." *The Routledge Companion to the Environmental Humanities*, edited by Ursula Heise et al., Routledge, 2017, pp. 222–31.
Willow, Anna. "Indigenous ExtrACTIVISM in Boreal Canada: Colonial Legacies, Contemporary Struggles and Sovereign Futures." *Humanities*, vol. 5, no. 3, July 2016, p. 55.
Yu, Ziwa, et al. "Characteristics of Indigenous Healing Strategies in Canada: A Scoping Review: A Scoping Review." *JBI Evidence Synthesis*, vol. 18, no. 12, Dec. 2020, pp. 2512–55.
Zanella, Patrizia. "Cherie Dimaline's *The Marrow Thieves*." *Studies in American Indian Literatures*, vol. 32, no. 3/4, 2020, pp. 176–200.

CONCLUSION

Illness as Genre

Physical trouble serves narrative ends. We have seen in the previous chapters how illness impacts social worlds, letting authors depict both selfless and corrupt relations between patients and caregivers and the circulation of potent information and drugs, as individual disorder flourishes into wider interpersonal conflict worth narrating. Throughout, the hope for cure offers a constant beacon. Illness thus gives structure and direction to narrative and so offers some of the benefits of genre to authors, who use its form to build progression in their stories.

Genre implies narrative trajectories, to marriage in romance and comedy, to death in tragedy. Illness too carries such vectors, whether the ultimate station is cure, mortality, or the changed reality of chronic ill-health. Illness also requires story to be known, and indeed practitioners use narrative to make diagnoses: they take the patient's history, then scan their mental catalogues of narrative forms to practise their trick of recognition by questioning what genre of story they have been told, which events conform and which do not, to arrive at a diagnosis.

I have aimed to observe illness within a canon of Canadian prose literature with an emphasis on novels, so I consider books that have drawn the attention of readers and critics and the institutional acclaim of awards. By examining this collection we can see how literary history, understood as past developments in writing and the life stories of celebrated authors, can inform notions of medical history, just as the history of medical science and knowledge can illuminate literature.

Intriguingly none of the works presented here focus on cancer, the leading cause of death according to Statistic Canada. This absence illustrates

DOI: 10.4324/9781003340119-7

the distance between literary narrative and purely documentary accounts of illness. Heart disease, the second most common ailment, also appears only tangentially in these works. Cancer and cardiac trouble may lack the social characteristics of more frequently narrated illnesses. For Susan Sontag the absence of cancer in popular discussion results from its perceived obscenity as a dark omen, and because "death is now an offensively meaningless event, so that disease widely considered a synonym for death is experienced as something to hide" (8). Yet, compared to many of the illnesses narrated in the books discussed here, cancer often originates without clear causes, without social contagion or spread, without any prospect of choice or narrative direction leading to it as an outcome, without allowing patients a sense of agency. The hope of cure seems inevitably in the hands of practitioners and their chemicals, whose banishments a tumour may or may not heed in a dance of consequence that the sufferer's own choices seem incapable of influencing. Likewise, the hypertension that often causes heart disease, stroke, and heart attack is known as a "silent killer," as the effects of decades of slowly accumulating choices may suddenly become clear—or the healthy lifestyles of marathon runners and careful eaters may still result in sudden death. Cancer and heart disease may not leave authors with as much scope for narration because of how they seem to deny rather than reveal individual agency.

If illness represents a genre, it is one that lets authors explore the agency of individuals in the face of their own and others' suffering. I have sought to illustrate how authors contend with suffering, its social consequences and challenges to communication, and many of these books query the extent to which language can express physical experiences of illness and pain. This habit of problematizing language may be a key benefit of reading literature for practitioners as they strive to interpret what their patients are saying alongside the signals of their bodies. Illness lets authors regard the limits of language and explore how the evidence of the body—its festering wounds, fever, and vomit—can communicate disorder beyond the abilities of words.

In fiction, this challenge of interpretation—the expression of the body contrasted with the words and stories a sick person may have to share—often transpires in a dramatized scene of care. Bedside scenes are spaces of frequently tense intersubjective communication, and we have seen how often an individual's illness impacts their interactions with others at many levels. Whereas epidemics change social relations at the scale of whole populations, the scene of medical care implies a much more intimate realm of social interaction. Like a stage, bedside scenes imply roles for characters—doctor, nurse, patient, family member—that they may or may not always wish to play, or that may mask or enable other identities and forms of authority—spy, prophet, matriarch. Throughout these scenes, information—from death-bed confessions, to gossip, to medical expertise—circulates between bodies like contagion.

Above all my concern has been with the relationship between illness and narrative. Narrative responds to disorder and uses the ordering velocity of language to create reason from the chaos of real experience. Disordered bodies give authors frames for their pursuit of this narrative work, as these chapters have explored. Illness shapes stories, starts and ends them, even as story can shape illness, can be a form of healing, and can make suffering knowable to loved ones, caregivers, wider national communities—and readers.

Works Cited

Sontag, Susan. *Illness as Metaphor*. Farrar, Straus and Giroux, 1978.

Statistics Canada. *Leading Causes of Death, Total Population, by Age Group*. Government of Canada, 27 Nov. 2023, www150.statcan.gc.ca/t1/tbl1/en/tv.action?pid=1310039401.

INDEX

FSC
www.fsc.org
MIX
Papier | Fördert gute Waldnutzung
FSC® C083411

Kolibri 360 GmbH
Ferdinand-Jühlke-Straße 7
99095 Erfurt, Deutschland
produktsicherheit@kolibri360.de